Chronic Obstructive
Pulmonary Disease

A Hazelden Pocket Health Guide

Chronic Obstructive Pulmonary Disease

Practical, Medical, and Spiritual Guidelines for Daily Living with Emphysema, Chronic Bronchitis, and Combination Diagnosis

MARK JENKINS

Foreword by Robert E. Larsen, M.D.

HAZELDEN

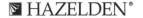

HAZELDEN®

INFORMATION & EDUCATIONAL SERVICES

Hazelden
Center City, Minnesota 55012-0176

1-800-328-0094
1-651-213-4590 (Fax)
www.hazelden.org

Library of Congress Cataloging-in-Publication Data

Jenkins, Mark, 1962–
    Chronic obstructive pulmonary disease : practical, medical, and
    spiritual guidelines for daily living with emphysema, chronic
    bronchitis, and combination diagnosis / Mark Jenkins ; foreword by
    Robert E. Larsen.
        p.   cm. — (A Hazelden pocket health guide)
    Includes bibliographical references and index.
    ISBN 1-56838-350-9
    1. Lungs—Diseases, Obstructive Popular works.   I. Title.
II. Series.
    RC776.09J46   1999
    616.2'4—dc21   99-35190
                                                                                  CIP

03 02 01 00 99   6 5 4 3 2 1

Editor's note
The excerpt from the book *Alcoholics Anonymous,* pages 83–84, and the
Twelve Steps are reprinted/adapted with permission of Alcoholics Anonymous
World Services, Inc. Permission to reprint pages 83–84 and the Twelve Steps
does not mean that AA has reviewed or approved the contents of this publication, or that AA necessarily agrees with the views expressed herein. AA is a
program of recovery from alcoholism *only*—use of pages 83–84 and the
Twelve Steps in connection with programs and activities which are patterned
after AA, but which address other problems, or in any other non-AA context,
does not imply otherwise.

Cover design by David Spohn
Interior design by Donna Burch
Typesetting by Stanton Publication Services, Inc.

Contents

Foreword

For the past sixty years, millions of addicts and alcoholics have stopped using drugs and found new, rewarding lives by following the spiritual principles outlined in Twelve Step programs such as Alcoholics Anonymous. From a medical perspective, it is not unreasonable to say that Twelve Step programs constitute the gold standard of treatment for the chronic disease of chemical dependency. These programs have been so successful that they are now used to deal with other challenges of a chronic nature, such as overeating, sexual compulsion, gambling, and depression.

The Hazelden Pocket Health Guide series is designed to help patients cope with chronic diseases, specifically, diseases that may be the result of an addiction. The long-term, potentially debilitating illnesses we refer to include chronic obstructive pulmonary disease (COPD), hypertension, and liver disease. This series can help patients make use of the same spiritual principles that have enabled so many chemically dependent people to lead full and satisfying lives.

Spirituality and acceptance are powerful tools patients and health care professionals can apply to help deal with disease. In thirty years of medical practice

I have seen many patients with chronic disease who, despite the best physicians and hospitals, have done poorly. Sometimes this was due to the severity of the disease process, but often, the patients' inability to accept the disease and its consequences was of significance. Denial is a common problem in chemically dependent people, but chemical dependency is by no means the only disease in which it plays a major role in the outcome. Denial is common to *every* chronic disease known to medical science and if not dealt with effectively is a major stumbling block to effective treatment.

Despite significant advances in treating diabetes, for instance, at least half of all diabetics fail to follow their diets or to take their medications properly. Many of these patients suffer amputations, kidney failure and dialysis, heart attacks, and blindness partly due to their disease but mostly due to the denial that blinds them to effective treatment of the disease.

Denial and chronic disease can be dealt with by using spiritual principles. Spirituality is not religion, although some people achieve it in traditional religious communities. Spirituality is the concept that each of us has a Higher Power that can help us cope with life. For many this is the traditional God, while for others it may be nature, the recovering community, or a set of guiding principles. Each person has his or her own concept of a Higher Power. Spirituality is not a particular religious dogma but rather a concept that allows people to feel good about how they live their lives.

Bill Wilson, the cofounder of Alcoholics Anonymous, described spirituality as the concept that we can do together what we could not do alone. Spirituality is about community and being a part of a greater whole. Spirituality is we *not* me.

Chronic Obstructive Pulmonary Disease (COPD)

Chronic obstructive pulmonary disease (COPD) affects millions of people worldwide every year. It is characterized by decreased lung function, chronic cough, shortness of breath, and wheezing. Left untreated, COPD can lead to death from heart failure or infection and pneumonia. Patients with COPD frequently find their daily activities curtailed due to difficulty in breathing. COPD is silent in its early years and usually manifests itself when its victims are in their forties and fifties. Unfortunately, many are not aware of this disease until it is too late to reverse its consequences.

The most common cause of COPD is cigarette smoking (nicotine addiction). While only 10 to 15 percent of smokers get COPD, the vast majority who have this disease are, or have been, moderate to heavy smokers. Other causes of COPD include asthma, environmental factors, and even a genetic defect. Smokers, however, are most commonly affected with COPD, and smoking cessation is absolutely critical in treating this condition.

COPD is a treatable disease, but it is not curable. Treatment, however, can be effective in slowing the disease and helping patients to live productive lives.

Spirituality will not make COPD go away. Using spiritual principles to complement medical therapy will help people cope with the disease. Dealing with denial and learning to coexist with the illness, instead of fighting it, are two of the goals of this work. If patients apply the principles found in these pages and cooperate with their health care providers' treatment plan, they will see an improvement in breathing and in overall quality of life. They will cease to fight the disease and in doing so will begin to know peace.

Robert E. Larsen, M.D.
Coordinator, Health Care Professionals Program
Hazelden Foundation

Preface

I owe my life to a spiritual program of recovery. My journey started when I joined the recovery community. By following the Twelve Steps of Alcoholics Anonymous (the basis of *all* Twelve Step programs), I found a new life. My career was rebuilt; my relationships with others were mended; my self-esteem was restored.

A natural-born cynic, I was at first astounded when so many of "the Promises" I had been told about came true—and in such short order (see pages xix–xx for more on the Promises). By then I had learned not to question but to simply accept such blessings as part of my continuing journey in sobriety.

As a medical writer with several books to my credit, I began to postulate that this spiritual program of recovery from addiction would be a revelation to people with chronic illnesses. After all, the Twelve Steps are a universal plan for living well. Countless groups apply the Twelve Steps to their addictions and conditions—everything ranging from Emotions Anonymous to Debtors Anonymous to Gamblers Anonymous to the grandparent of them all, Alcoholics Anonymous. And so I set about writing a book that offers a spiritual program of recovery from chronic illness.

Probably no one needs a guide to living well more than people who suffer from long-term medical conditions that dominate their lives. Chronic illness affects more than ninety million Americans and, according to the American Medical Association, is this nation's foremost health concern. Chronic illness leads to feelings of anger, isolation and loneliness, financial difficulties, compromised personal relationships, and trouble at work. The emotional consequences of a chronic illness are especially profound when the condition is caused by a dependency on a mood-altering substance such as nicotine or alcohol. The Twelve Step program helps people deal with these overwhelming emotions by teaching them how to find their spirituality.

I am hardly the first person to suggest that the Twelve Steps can benefit those with chronic illnesses. Many others whose lives have been transformed by a Twelve Step program have applied these principles to conditions ranging from cancer to AIDS.

However, what has been lacking in these interpretations is a plan for individual conditions. Until now.

This book is part of the Hazelden Pocket Health Guide series of books that adapts the Twelve Steps for those with chronic illnesses—in this case, chronic obstructive pulmonary disease. The book combines specific medical guidelines with a plan to improve emotional and spiritual well-being. At its core is a program of hope, happiness, and healing.

Above all, this program provides those with chronic illnesses like COPD what they need: the indispensable tools and inspiration to live life one day at a time . . . and to *live it well.*

Spirituality:
The Strongest Medicine of All?

Can spirituality help me beat my disease? That's probably the question you're asking yourself. A better question might be, Can the spiritual program this book teaches help me overcome the emotional pain of my disease so I can manage my disease more effectively? The answer to that question is "yes."

A growing body of evidence suggests that spirituality actually helps us stay healthy and recover from illness. How? For a quarter-century doctors have wondered the same thing—and now believe they know the answer. Researchers at Harvard's Mind/Body Medical Institute found in extensive laboratory studies that prayer and meditation—prerequisites for a sound spiritual life—cause a person's body to undergo healthful changes.[1] There is decreased metabolism, heart rate, and rate of breathing, as well as slower brain waves. These changes are the opposite of those induced by stress and are an effective therapy for chronic illnesses. In fact, doctors like those at the Mind/Body

1. For a brochure describing the Mind/Body Medical Institute, call (617) 632-9525 or visit its Web site at www.mindbody.harvard.edu

Medical Institute believe that a spiritual program that involves prayer and meditation is an effective component of treatment for any disease made worse by stress.

Although skeptics still question whether a spiritual person is more likely to recover from chronic illness than one who is not, of this there is no doubt: spirituality helps chronically ill people cope with the emotional challenges of their condition.

But just what is spirituality anyway? One thing it *isn't* is religion. Although many truly religious people are spiritual, and many spiritual people consider themselves religious, the two concepts are not one and the same. You don't have to be religious to be spiritual. Religion is a formalization of society's relationship with God into rituals and institutions. Spirituality is our inherent belief in the existence of a higher power, energy, or force—or what is perceived as God—and a feeling of closeness to that entity.

That being is referred to variously within these pages as a Higher Power, a Power greater than ourselves, or Power Greater.

This book advocates the use of the Twelve Steps, a spiritual program founded in the 1930s to help alcoholics recover from the disease of alcoholism. The Twelve Steps can help you "turn over" care of your disease to a Higher Power that is greater than you, that is wiser than you, and that loves you. And it will help you maintain strength and hope as you live each day with your disease.

You'll learn in depth about the Twelve Steps later in this book. Right now what's important is that you know that recovery from chronic obstructive pulmonary disease (usually known by its acronym, COPD) isn't just about addressing the medical aspects of the disease, although you will certainly learn most of what you need to know in these pages. No, recovery from COPD is also about learning to overcome the emotional pain of chronic illness. Only by doing this will you be able to properly manage your disease.

The Twelve Steps will help you overcome your emotional pain by allowing you to recognize what you do and don't have control over. In cooperation with your Higher Power, you have the power to deal with your feelings about your disease and to change the behaviors that caused or exacerbated the condition. You can also take those all-important steps to prevent it from getting worse, such as taking your medication, exercising, avoiding dangerous environments, and, above all, resisting the urge to smoke. The Twelve Steps will also show you how to grow spiritually through prayer and meditation, making amends to others, and spending time in the company of other people with COPD.

There is no cure for COPD, just as there is no cure

for alcoholism and other chronic illnesses. However, the Twelve Steps have provided those who have practiced the principles of the program with the life skills they need to live immensely fulfilling lives—in many respects, the kind of spiritual lives they would never have had the opportunity to experience had they not developed a chronic illness.

Despite their popularity, Twelve Step programs are still widely misunderstood in some quarters. Such misunderstandings stand in the way of acceptance by those who could really use them, including people with chronic illnesses such as COPD. Perhaps the most common misunderstanding is that Twelve Step programs are "covers" for religion—specifically, Christian groups.

A hasty reading of the Steps may reinforce this impression. However, after reading more carefully, people soon discover that the Steps do not endorse any religion. A person who lives by the Steps could be Jewish, Christian, Hindu, Muslim, Buddhist, agnostic, or atheist.

If the Twelve Steps are not a religious program, then they certainly are a spiritual one. The Steps echo what writer Aldous Huxley called the "perennial philosophy"—a core set of ideas and practices shared by many religious traditions. The Steps have one major concern, and that is human transformation.

Many of you may already be intimately familiar with a Twelve Step program. Those of you who aren't will discover that it offers a new approach to living. This approach is available to you if you acknowledge your jeopardy and your need to learn to change your behaviors and to improve your state of being.

The spiritual component of this book draws extensively on principles developed by the founders of Alcoholics Anonymous. Like alcoholism, COPD is a chronic disease that is always with its sufferers to some degree and affects every area of their lives. The extraordinary success achieved by millions of "AAs" can be emulated by those with COPD who follow the Steps suggested in this book.

It is heartening to know that the same Promises which inspire Alcoholics Anonymous members also offer strength and hope to those with COPD who are willing to follow this simple program:

> If we are painstaking about this phase of our development, we will be amazed before we are half way through. We are going to know a new freedom and a new happiness. We will not regret the past nor wish to shut the door on it. We will comprehend the word serenity and we will know peace. No matter how far down the scale we have gone, we will see how our experience can benefit others. That feeling of uselessness and self-pity

will disappear. We will lose interest in selfish things and gain interest in our fellows. Self-seeking will slip away. Our whole attitude and outlook upon life will change. Fear of people and of economic insecurity will leave us. We will intuitively know how to handle situations which used to baffle us. We will suddenly realize that God is doing for us what we could not do for ourselves.[2]

The Twelve Step program of spirituality discussed in this book emphasizes acceptance. Most health care professionals would probably agree—it is only when you accept that you have COPD that you can take the steps necessary to address it. Thus the first part of this book describes the chronic disease of COPD, its physical and psychological symptoms, its causes, and its treatment.

The Twelve Steps for COPD[3]

Step One—We admitted we were powerless over chronic illness—that our lives had become unmanageable.

Step Two—Came to believe that a Power greater than ourselves could restore us to sanity.

Step Three—Made a decision to turn our will

---

2. *Alcoholics Anonymous,* 3d. ed. (New York: Alcoholics Anonymous World Services, Inc., 1976), 83–84. Reprinted with permission.

3. Adapted from the Twelve Steps of Alcoholics Anonymous with the permission of AA World Services, Inc., New York, N.Y.

and our lives over to the care of a Power greater than ourselves.

Step Four—Made a searching and fearless moral inventory of ourselves.

Step Five—Admitted to the God of our understanding, to ourselves, and to another human being the exact nature of our wrongs.

Step Six—Were entirely ready to have the God of our understanding remove all these defects of character.

Step Seven—Humbly asked our Higher Power to remove our shortcomings.

Step Eight—Made a list of all persons we had harmed and became willing to make amends to them all.

Step Nine—Made direct amends to such people wherever possible, except when to do so would injure them or others.

Step Ten—Continued to take personal inventory and when we were wrong promptly admitted it.

Step Eleven—Sought through prayer and meditation to improve our conscious contact with a Power greater than ourselves, praying only for knowledge of our Higher Power's will and the courage to carry that out.

Step Twelve—Having had a spiritual awakening as the result of these steps, we tried to carry our message to others with our condition and to practice these principles in all our affairs.

The Twelve Steps of Alcoholics Anonymous[4]

Step One—We admitted we were powerless over alcohol—that our lives had become unmanageable.

Step Two—Came to believe that a Power greater than ourselves could restore us to sanity.

Step Three—Made a decision to turn our will and our lives over to the care of God *as we understood Him.*

Step Four—Made a searching and fearless moral inventory of ourselves.

Step Five—Admitted to God, to ourselves, and to another human being the exact nature of our wrongs.

Step Six—Were entirely ready to have God remove all these defects of character.

Step Seven—Humbly asked Him to remove our shortcomings.

Step Eight—Made a list of all persons we had harmed, and became willing to make amends to them all.

---

4. The Twelve Steps of AA are taken from *Alcoholics Anonymous,* 3d ed., published by AA World Services, Inc., New York, N.Y., 59–60. Reprinted with permission of AA World Services, Inc. (See editor's note on copyright page.)

Step Nine—Made direct amends to such people wherever possible, except when to do so would injure them or others.

Step Ten—Continued to take personal inventory and when we were wrong promptly admitted it.

Step Eleven—Sought through prayer and meditation to improve our conscious contact with God *as we understood Him,* praying only for knowledge of His will for us and the power to carry that out.

Step Twelve—Having had a spiritual awakening as the result of these steps, we tried to carry this message to alcoholics, and to practice these principles in all our affairs.

CHAPTER ONE

COPD Essentials

What Is COPD?

Chronic obstructive pulmonary disease (COPD) is an umbrella term for a variety of lung disorders whose symptoms may at first seem quite mild but eventually compromise every aspect of life. Unless treated, a person with COPD will inevitably suffer life-threatening enlargement of the heart and heart failure *(cor pulmonale)* caused by the strain of breathing problems. The consequences of COPD aren't just physical. As with any debilitating chronic illness, the emotional and psychological repercussions can be devastating.

Occupational hazards such as microscopic airborne debris may occasionally cause COPD. The condition is also associated with a rare congenital deficiency of the protein antitrypsin. However, research shows that *a full 80 to 90 percent of COPD cases are caused by smoking tobacco.*

Approximately twenty-five million Americans have

COPD, and it is the fifth leading cause of death in the United States. Significantly, COPD diagnoses have increased dramatically—by an astounding 60 percent—between 1982 and 1994. The number of lives claimed by COPD has increased sharply too. In 1979, COPD accounted for about 50,000 deaths. In 1982, the number rose to 59,000, and by 1994, the number of deaths attributed to COPD reached 96,000.

More men than women have COPD because, until recently, more men than women were heavy smokers. The average American with COPD is sixty-five years old and has a long history of smoking.[1]

Just What Does Chronic Obstructive Pulmonary Disease Mean?

Chronic—Refers to a continual, permanent, incurable condition that affects all aspects of life.

Obstructive—To block or fill.

Pulmonary—Of or pertaining to the lungs.

Disease—A condition with signs and symptoms that have profound emotional consequences.

---

1. Typically, people who develop COPD have a smoking history of over ten "pack-years." The term "pack-years" refers to the total amount of smoking over a lifetime. Ten pack-years can mean a pack a day for ten years, two packs a day for five years, or half a pack a day for twenty years.

Symptoms of COPD

The characteristic symptoms of COPD are shortness of breath accompanied by wheezing, dark-colored phlegm, and a chronic cough.

Do you have COPD? Ask yourself the following questions:

- Am I a longtime heavy smoker? Or was I at one time?
- Do I often experience shortness of breath?
- Do I have frequent bouts of what seems to be bronchitis?
- When I catch a cold, does it last weeks instead of days?
- Do I have a morning "smoker's cough"?
- Do I cough up greenish-yellow phlegm?
- Do I experience coughing fits during exertions as mild as climbing the stairs or carrying groceries?

If you answered "yes" to two or more of the above questions and are a longtime heavy smoker (or used to be) who is over forty years of age, you may have COPD. See a doctor.

Symptoms Table

Severity of COPD	When chronic bronchitis dominates	When emphysema dominates
MILD	* Coughing with phlegm for more than three months at a time for two consecutive years	* Possibly no early signs/symptoms
MODERATE	* Shortness of breath from moderate exertion * Coughing and increased phlegm * Recurrent chest infections or bronchitis	* Shortness of breath from moderate exertion
SEVERE	* Severe shortness of breath * Coughing and excessive phlegm * Wheezing * Recurrent infections * Fluid buildup (esp. at the ankles) and bluish skin color	* Severe shortness of breath * Barrel-shaped chest

Causes of COPD

COPD is the result of repetitive damage to the lungs and is almost always caused by years of smoking. About 10 to 15 percent of all heavy smokers develop COPD. It is not known why some heavy smokers develop COPD while others do not.

The risk of a heavy smoker developing COPD increases when he or she is exposed to severe industrial air pollution on a regular basis (e.g., living or growing up in an area where there are a large number of factories). Air pollution, however, is not thought to be a sole cause of COPD.

Though rare, other causes of COPD include occupational hazards such as chemical fumes and dusts from grain, cotton, wood, or mining by-products. And, as stated earlier, in very few cases emphysema-related COPD is caused by an inherited lack of the protein antitrypsin.

Diagnosing COPD

The earlier you determine you have COPD and take steps to control it, the better. You will be able to reduce its symptoms, prevent infections, and lead a more active life. Regrettably, by the time most people with COPD seek medical attention, the damage has been done.

SEE A DOCTOR!

People often seek help too late, after extensive damage to the lungs has already taken place. Although a precise diagnosis can be difficult to make, the best way for your doctor to determine whether you have COPD is by taking a complete medical history and performing a spirometry test.

Medical History

In the medical history, your doctor will ask you many of those same questions you asked yourself on page 3 concerning your smoking and current health.

Spirometry Test

Spirometry is the most reliable method of testing lung health. The name of this test refers to the machine used to perform the test, the spirometer. You blow into a tube attached to the spirometer, and it measures how long it takes you to empty your lungs of air and how much air you managed to exhale. The more damaged your lungs, the less air you will be able to blow out, and the longer it will take.

If the spirometry test reveals you have breathing problems, your doctor may want to know how well your lungs exchange oxygen for carbon dioxide (a waste gas you exhale). This involves taking blood from an artery to find out how much oxygen it contains.

COPD: A Progressive Disease

COPD causes a gradual but inevitable decline in lung function. In the beginning there may be few symptoms, while in the final stages of COPD there is severe shortness of breath, frequent coughing, excessive amount of phlegm, and painful infections. These symptoms interfere with almost every aspect of life, even the simple act of sleeping.

Anatomy of a Disease

COPD usually refers to a combination of two conditions—*chronic bronchitis* and *emphysema*. Both these conditions involve lung damage. Here's how that damage occurs.

Chronic Bronchitis

Many people develop bronchitis at one time or another but experience only temporary symptoms: a bad cough, trouble breathing, and excessive production of yellowish-green phlegm. If you have COPD with a bronchitis component, however, these symptoms last months, not days or weeks. If the disease has progressed, the symptoms may be present all the time.

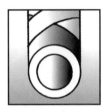

Healthy Airway

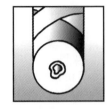

Airway with
Chronic Bronchitis

Chronic bronchitis principally affects the vast complex of air passages *(bronchi)* that connect the windpipe *(trachea)* in your throat to the tiny air sacs *(alveoli)* deep in your lungs. If you have chronic bronchitis, the bronchi have been irritated, most likely by years of smoking. As a result, the walls of these tubes swell up, narrowing the airways and making it difficult for air to pass through. Although a certain amount of phlegm is necessary, irritated bronchi produce an excess of this gooey substance, which not only contributes to the blockage but also provides a fertile ground for infections.

Emphysema

If you have emphysema, the damage is to the tiny air sacs *(alveoli)* at the ends of the air passages *(bronchi)* that reach deep into your lungs.

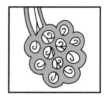

Healthy Air Sacs

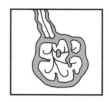

Air Sacs in a Person
with Emphysema

Due to blockage of these airways as pictured above, air has difficulty reaching the air sacs and then being let out of them through the airways. As a result of this dysfunction, the walls of your air sacs get damaged: they stretch out, become less pliable, and eventually break down. This process makes your lungs larger and less efficient at doing the job of exchanging oxygen for carbon dioxide, which makes breathing difficult.

Treatment of COPD can reduce symptoms, help prevent infections, and permit a more active lifestyle. Younger people with COPD have a better prognosis than older people. Unfortunately, by the time a person suffering from COPD has symptoms severe enough that they seek treatment, the damage to the lungs is already done. In such cases, life expectancy is significantly curtailed, and quality of life suffers immeasurably.

COPD has been dubbed "the silent killer" because

its deadly symptoms inexorably worsen without you being aware of it. In the beginning you may notice some shortness of breath when you're climbing the stairs or carrying groceries to the car. Then you start to develop an irritating "smoker's cough." At first the symptoms may not seem serious, and with time, you may adjust to them. Inevitably, though, your symptoms deteriorate to where even the simplest everyday tasks become a major effort that leave you out of breath: dressing, doing laundry, even eating.

In addition to causing severe medical symptoms, like any chronic illness, COPD has emotional and psychological consequences too. Most people diagnosed with COPD experience anger, frustration, depression, anxiety, and feelings of worthlessness as their condition worsens.

COPD cannot be cured, but it can be contained. The earlier in its progression COPD is detected and the more assertively a COPD sufferer addresses his or her condition, the more effective the treatment will be.

Components of a successful program to address the progression of COPD and the severity of its physical and psychological symptoms include the following:

• Get the right medical attention.
• Enter a comprehensive rehabilitation program.
• Join a support group.

- Make lifestyle changes, especially smoking cessation.
- Prevent or treat lung infection.
- Take medicine properly.
- Reduce exposure to environmental hazards.
- Adopt strategies for daily activities.
- Work on your spirituality.

COPD: The Mind-Body Connection

The symptoms of COPD aren't just physical; they are emotional and psychological too. Feelings of low self-esteem, guilt, and frustration may be exacerbated because COPD is often caused by addictive behavior. Addressing these emotional and psychological components of the disease is integral to treating COPD as a whole. Improved mental health helps us cope with the physical challenges of our disease, hence the phrase "mind-body connection."

Powerful evidence suggests that practicing the principles of a spiritual program will enhance people's ability to cope emotionally and psychologically with conditions like COPD.

The medical profession is at last coming to recognize the need for a spiritual component in the management of chronic illnesses. Most doctors who deal with chronically ill people understand the benefits of support groups, whether or not they are spiritual in nature.

Gradually, the medical profession is beginning to acknowledge the great gift that is available to those people with chronic illness who commit to exploring their spirituality.

Sometimes I Feel Like Crying[2]

At some point in a Wellness Program, and in some Rehabilitation Programs, someone will address the subject of "stress." When that person addresses a group of COPD patients, I feel it would be far better to drop the euphemisms and talk openly and candidly about the fear, depression, anger, resentment, frustration, and loss of self-esteem most of us struggle with at one time or another, and teach us that success in coping with these emotions may well be the single most important element in the management of our disease.

Few medical professionals know, firsthand, the frustration of being so short of breath you can barely make it to the bathroom and back, or how difficult it may be to towel-off after a bath, or how it feels to be dependent upon a little plastic tube you must wear in your nose and drag behind you everywhere you go. And I bet they can't imagine how tears come to your eyes

---

2. Excerpted with permission from *A COPD Survival Guide,* copyright 1997 by Bill Horden.

when you remember the way you used to get your work done in an orderly fashion and reasonable time, or how well you bowled or played softball, or the last time you danced across the floor with your spouse or grandchild in your arms. Do they understand that you can't breathe when you lie down, so you must spend your nights in a chair; and what it's like to now need from others the help you were always the first to offer to them?

Luckily, most people have been spared the feeling that comes with the closing-off of your throat that makes you clutch your breast and gasp for breath and fumble for an inhaler, and the mounting fear that compounds the problem, as you anticipate it getting worse . . . so bad you may be in the hospital emergency room . . . again.

I could expand on this by mentioning the deep depression that causes some patients to give up on their therapy or quit (or conveniently "forget" their medications, or the problem of self-esteem (or vanity) that keeps some patients from taking needed medications, or using their oxygen units in public. And I could address the many times a patient asks his God, "Why me?" But I think I've made my point.

The Psychological Impact of COPD

The psychological impact of a debilitating chronic illness can be as devastating for someone with COPD as the physical symptoms. These psychological symptoms, which may occur quite apart from the symptoms of the disease itself, are commonly associated with COPD:

- *profound, persistent episodes of sadness lasting for longer than two weeks*
- *loss of interest in favorite activities*
- *difficulty sleeping*
- *feeling depressed most of the day*
- *decreased sexual drive*
- *feelings of worthlessness*
- *difficulty concentrating*
- *absentmindedness*
- *recurrent thoughts of suicide*

The potential severity of these symptoms reinforces the need for health care for COPD sufferers that goes beyond medical treatment. Doctors often recommend that people with these symptoms seek help from a mental health professional, such as a therapist, and join a support group where members can share common experiences and problems.

CHAPTER TWO

A Spiritual Program for Transcending the Emotional Pain of COPD

Anger, shame, resentment, fear, and despondency—these are all emotions you may have experienced when you discovered you had COPD. Feelings of anguish such as these are common—even expected—when you face the reality of your disease and the harsh consequences of a smoking addiction.

When you first find out you have COPD, your first instinct may be to lash out. Or you may find yourself wanting to withdraw from the world at large. Some of you will do both—retreat from society and assail those who dare to encroach upon your isolation.

The despair that may cause you to lose interest in your own welfare is especially pernicious when you have COPD. Successfully containing the physical symptoms of COPD requires assiduous effort on your part. Yet the tendency at first may be to "give up on life." Dealing with it all feels overwhelming.

Neglecting medical treatment because of emotional distress creates a self-perpetuating cycle of physical and emotional deterioration, a downward spiral of disability and depression that inevitably leads to early death.

But it doesn't have to be that way.

The good news is that having a chronic illness presents you with the opportunity to change yourself *for the better.* Most people want to improve themselves; but for you, this desire holds the promise of even greater rewards. Yes, you have been stricken with a potentially devastating chronic illness, but you can nevertheless learn to live a life that is happy, joyous, and free—a life that may even be better than ever.

The question is, how do you go about this?

To achieve the serenity and acceptance you need to cope successfully with your disease, you need a spiritual plan as well as a medical one. The Twelve Step program referred to throughout this book has worked with astonishing success for millions of people with the chronic illnesses of addiction, including alcoholism and other drug addictions, gambling, and overeating. Its principles have also provided great succor for people with other chronic illnesses.

The Twelve Step program is, at its core, spiritual. It is strictly nondenominational, however, and accommodates people of all faiths. The program also welcomes those who do not have religious faith. Nevertheless, success in this program requires a profound change in thinking from self-centeredness to one that accepts the role of a "Higher Power."

How you see your Higher Power is a matter of personal choice. It does not have to be "God" in a traditional sense. Although some people do turn to a God as their Higher Power, others receive spiritual direction from their support groups, the Twelve Steps themselves, or another source. More important than your definition of a Higher Power is that you work with that Power and remain open to its influence.

Thanks to the foresight of those who created the Twelve Step program, this guide to better living with chronic illness is flexibile. This set of principles makes no draconian demands on you but rather offers suggestions for behavior that will result in an improved life with less emotional pain and greater spiritual living.

There is no rule about how the Steps should be done; this is a matter of personal preference. Many people with chronic illness have experienced great improvement in their spiritual well-being by choosing to do the Steps selectively. However, the Steps exist in the order described because those who have followed them in sequence have found they work best that way. The Twelve Steps build on each other. You get a firm foothold on one Step before you go on to the next. To follow the Steps in this order is to journey from acceptance to serenity one Step at a time.

Many people ask if there is a time frame for doing the Steps. "As long as it takes" is probably the best advice. But it is important to feel you are making progress. If possible, you don't want to feel stalled on one Step or take lengthy breaks between them.

And keep in mind that doing the Steps isn't a one-time thing. You continue to practice the principles of the Steps in your daily life, and there is nothing to stop you from starting again on Step One and working all the way to Step Twelve whenever you wish. For many people, "working the Steps" provides tremendous serenity and satisfaction, not to mention a simple plan for living well.

A careful reading of this part of the book will reveal that the underlying concepts of the Twelve Steps are not unique. Those who developed the Twelve Steps simply wrote a book about how they got sober. But the steps they took are supported by the collective sagacity of philosophers and religious leaders from different cultures throughout the ages. You will soon see that the message in the Steps is ageless; the philosophy is timeless; and the strength and hope offered to those with chronic illnesses like COPD is everlasting.

Much has been written about the Twelve Steps. The following pages will introduce you to each Step. If this is your first encounter with the Steps, you may find it helpful to gather more information. If you've been exposed to the Steps or currently work the program for an addiction, this chapter can serve as a review.

Step One: The Foundation of Recovery

We admitted we were powerless over chronic illness—that our lives had become unmanageable.

We've probably all heard it said that the first step is the hardest to take. This is certainly true with the Twelve Steps. In taking Step One, we must admit to being powerless over whether we have COPD and recognize that our lives are out of control. Who wants to do such a thing? Step One gets us to face reality—we cannot alter the fact that we have COPD. We suffer from a disease that is *incurable.* Not only that, but it is starting to affect our lives in very distressing ways. We cough, wheeze, and gasp through another day. Our families fret. There are arguments about going to see the doctor, taking medication, not smoking. For years we told ourselves things weren't so bad, yet try as we might to deny it, we knew inside there was something very, very wrong with our health.

The First Step takes courage. It means accepting

that having this disease is out of our hands. Believing otherwise makes our lives unmanageable. Acceptance is the turning point for change. Unless we accept our disease, we cannot move forward. Like thousands who have gone before us, we can summon the courage we need to take this Step, the first in our spiritual journey toward achieving the serenity we need to manage our disease in its entirety.

Step Two: A Promise of Hope

Came to believe that a Power greater than ourselves could restore us to sanity.

At this time in our lives—having just been diagnosed with an incurable illness that we know will end our lives prematurely—many of us feel anything but kindly disposed to things spiritual. But spirituality is an integral part of any Twelve Step program for chronic illness. Why? Because to find the serenity and strength we need to manage this disease, we need to find a Power beyond ourselves.

Many of us already believe in a Higher Power we call God—though our faith may have been sorely tested by finding out we have COPD. If we don't have a belief in a Power greater than ourselves, it's important we at least stay open-minded about the concept. Even the slightest amount of faith that a Higher Power can and will help us is better than no faith at all. If this proves difficult, we "act as if" we believe, so we're open to experiencing its power.

Indeed, Step Two does not mean we must immediately come to believe in God in the traditional sense or in the context of formal religion. If we think this is the case, we dismiss the Twelve Step program because we think it won't work for us. Or, if we are religious, we may view the Steps as some sort of cult. We need to keep an open mind. Like all the Steps, Step Two is a suggestion from others who say, "This is the way it worked for us." Such people have found that the Second Step gave them hope—and there is hope for us, too, if we come to believe that the source of power we need lies outside ourselves.

If we were to ask all the COPD sufferers who have been restored to sanity how they identify their Higher Power, we would probably hear answers as varied as humankind's ideas about faith. Some might say God as they understand Him from the faith of their upbringing (the Christian God, for example); others could say God working through the Twelve Step program; while still more might say their Power Greater was the Twelve Steps themselves and support group attendance and fellowship. They would undoubtedly tell us that their relationship with their Higher Power helped them to step outside themselves and realize they were not the center of the universe.

Step Three: Turning It Over

Made a decision to turn our will and our lives over to the care of a Power greater than ourselves.

Of all the Steps, the Third Step can be the most effective in helping us transcend the emotional pain of chronic illness. Time and time again Step Three has provided what people needed to get through difficult moments and has helped them approach the management of their disease with remarkable resolve.

In Step One we admitted we were powerless over the fact that we have COPD and that our disease had made our lives unmanageable. In Step Two we came to believe that a Higher Power could help us get through our emotional pain. In Step Three we make the decision to let our Higher Power relieve us from the emotional pain and unmanageability of our disease and show us what we can do ourselves.

Turning our will over to a Power greater than ourselves doesn't absolve us from doing whatever is necessary to care for ourselves. Our Higher Power loves us whatever we do and helps us best by showing us how to help ourselves. Our Higher Power speaks through others and through us. We learn to listen to our feelings and to act on them.

No longer will we try to force impossible solutions or beliefs that aren't in our best interest. We won't expend time and energy "willing" our disease to go away. We let our Higher Power determine the best way for us to handle our disease and all the emotions that go along with it.

It is the responsibility of each and every one of us with COPD to cooperate with our Higher Power. We need to do all that we can to make ourselves physically and psychologically better—by taking our medicines regularly, exercising and eating properly, avoiding substances that we know are harmful to us, spending time in the company of others, and helping those sicker than we are.

Turning our will and our lives over to the care of a Higher Power doesn't "cure" our COPD or prevent our symptoms from getting worse. It doesn't stop us from having really bad days. But it does help us handle these challenges better. It gives us the ability to consider a plan or purpose higher than our own.

Achieving the balance between letting our Higher Power care for us and taking personal responsibility can be hard. We discover how to achieve this balance by communicating with our Higher Power through prayer and meditation. In this way the answers are often revealed.

Once we have begun the process of "turning it

over," we can begin to find relief from the emotional pain caused by our COPD. We can halt, go inside ourselves, and in the tranquillity simply say the Serenity Prayer: "'God, grant me the serenity to accept the things I cannot change, the courage to change the things I can, and the wisdom to know the difference.' Thy will, not mine, be done."

Can I be spiritual if I am not religious? Yes. You don't have to be religious to be spiritual. Being spiritual means believing in the existence of a Higher Power and feeling close to that Power; it does not necessarily mean believing in "God" in a traditional sense. People who are spiritual accept that they are not in control of their lives and trust that their Higher Power will take care of them.

Step Four: Knowing Yourself

Made a searching and fearless moral inventory of ourselves.

The importance of doing an inventory is to know ourselves better. By being searching and fearless about our liabilities, we gain an improved insight into how it was we came to develop the disease COPD and why it is we react the way we do. Writing down our inventory helps us to clearly understand what we need to do to correct the behaviors that brought us to this point and which ways of living will best help us manage our disease.

In doing this Step we must be *moral* but not *moralistic*. Our behavior has been good and bad—that is the reality. We must examine it. Make it ours. For example, most of us smoked for many years. Not only was that self-destructive, it was selfish and egotistical too. We ignored other people's desire not to be exposed to our secondhand smoke; we hurt our physical being; we used nicotine to numb feelings, stunting our emotional development. Self-centeredness was our credo because we would do anything to continue smoking.

What about pride? We refused for a long time to admit that the wheezing, coughing, and breathlessness meant we were sick. We also need to examine our behavior since being diagnosed with COPD. Have we indulged in excessive self-pity and ignored our doctors' recommendations? Have we taken our frustrations and anger out on our family and friends? Do we continue to smoke?

We mustn't punish ourselves for these things. The goal is to know ourselves and to accept ourselves. Only when we see ourselves in a way that is enlightening, not judgmental, can we strive to do better.

There are several ways to go about Step Four. The

most common way is to use a straightforward, double-column list of specific positive and negative behaviors.

Keep in mind that Step Four is not a test; we cannot fail it.

Taking the Fourth Step is a profound yet simple start to an ongoing way of daily living. It is the beginning of a path to self-awareness, a way to go today and each day hereafter. The inventory becomes a way of life based on the courage and willingness to be completely honest to oneself about oneself.

This self-assessment may be the most difficult feat of your life. If you need encouragement, support, or help, ask for it from someone you trust, such as a chaplain or counselor—someone who will be non-judgmental.

When we have completed our Fourth Step inventories, we will possess more self-awareness and self-acceptance. We're now ready for the Fifth Step. We're now ready to make some changes in our lives and in the ways we manage our disease.

Step Five: Telling My Story

Admitted to the God of our understanding, to ourselves, and to another human being the exact nature of our wrongs.

In the Fifth Step we openly, honestly, and willingly share who we are. This is a time for introspection as well as for laying ourselves bare. It allows us to let our Higher Power and another person see us for who we really are—flawed but lovable people who really *are* worthy of freedom from the emotional pain of our chronic illness.

Step Five gives us the chance to rid ourselves of the hidden side of ourselves, the side that sometimes causes us to feel shame.

We need to prepare for this Step. True self-awareness and honesty do not come easily to most people. We are used to avoiding our character defects. To stand and actually face ourselves as we truly are is a difficult and spiritually demanding proposition.

The key to a good Step Five is to have done a thorough, balanced, and honest Fourth Step. In particular, the kind of rigorous self-honesty called for in Step Four helps us to gain the *humility* we need to do an effective Step Five.

To Admit to a Higher Power

With the help of a Higher Power, we can find the inner courage and strength we need to take the Fifth Step. Caring, loving, and forgiving, our Higher Power will help us realize that we are not the only ones who fall short.

To Admit to Ourselves

To admit to ourselves where we went wrong is a sign that we are practicing true self-honesty. But it isn't easy. Who wants to confess to themselves the character flaws that may have caused them to develop a chronic illness? We go through our lives ignoring the ways we inflicted damage on our own bodies. Really, though, we do not forget. The knowledge gnaws at us.

Taking the Fifth Step without being totally self-honest is self-defeating and merely perpetuates our feeling of self-dishonesty.

To do this Step well, it is important to love and respect ourselves. Step Five allows us to reflect on the ways we are coping with our disease in a loving and nonjudgmental manner. It gives us the chance to accept ourselves as flawed human beings. It lets us understand that we need forgiveness and another chance at life. When we forgive ourselves, we are freed from the grip of guilt and shame.

To admit first to ourselves before admitting to another person shows we are willing to be really honest. We prove we are not afraid to face our real selves squarely. Knowing ourselves and our strengths and weaknesses intimately can profoundly help us transcend the emotional pain of a nicotine addiction and our COPD.

To Admit to Another Person

We share the Fifth Step with another person. Why? Because sharing with another person the exact nature of our wrongs keeps us honest. By doing this Step we allow another person to see us as complete, but flawed, human beings.

However, most of us will find this to be the hardest part of the Fifth Step. There is the overwhelming fear of embarrassment. Yet it is precisely the nature of these wrongs that makes them so important to discard.

Step Five is the opportunity to "cast out" those behaviors and traits that are causing us emotional pain. The wisdom of so many who have gone before us tells us that it is not enough merely to acknowledge the nature of our wrongs to ourselves and through prayer to a Higher Power. It is only by speaking out, admitting out loud our mistakes, failures, and anxieties to another person, that the power of those feelings and deeds loses its control over us. For those of us with a chronic illness like COPD, the Fifth Step is one major step away from a sense of isolation and loneliness and a step toward wholeness, happiness, and a real sense of gratitude.

Which "Human Being"?

During Step Five, most people wonder who they should share their secrets with. The fact is that almost anyone will do—a clergy person, a doctor, a psychologist, a family member who won't be adversely affected by your total honesty, a counselor, a friend, or even a stranger. There are, however, certain qualities that make a person a good candidate:

- *discretion*
- *maturity and wisdom*
- *willingness to share his or her own experiences*
- *familiarity with the challenges of a chronic illness*

Often, such people are not readily available to us. One of our responsibilities in doing the Fifth Step is to look around carefully for someone who meets these criteria.

Whomever we decide to share our Fifth Step with, remember that our intention is not to please that person but to heal ourselves. It is our inner selves we are trying to satisfy. We should also not be afraid of shocking listeners with our revelations.

Steps Four and Five Are Ongoing

The "housecleaning" process we do in Steps Four and Five is not meant to be a onetime event.

As we will learn in Step Ten, regular personal inventories are measures we can take to help us transcend the emotional pain of our chronic disease and better manage our condition. If and when we decide to do these Steps again, we remember that we do not need to go back over our whole lives but need only pick up where we left off when we last took inventory and admitted where we went wrong. What is past is past. What has been acknowledged once need not be discussed again, unless certain incidents or feelings have recurred or a pattern of behavior we overlooked has recently been detected. Whenever we take another Fourth and Fifth Step, it can become an opportunity for increasing our self-knowledge and self-acceptance, and for learning to forgive and seek forgiveness as a way of daily living.

Step Six: Ready, Willing, and Able

Were entirely ready to have the God of our understanding remove all these defects of character.

In Step One we admitted we were powerless over our disease. In Step Two we came to believe that our Higher Power could help us. In Step Three we made the decision to let that Power care for our lives. Steps Four and Five uncovered our defects of character.

If we have done these first five Steps honestly and

thoroughly, we will be ready to let go of our character defects. The *readiness* to have them removed is the key to the Sixth Step. By being willing to let go of these character defects, we increase our chances of being able to cope with our COPD.

In taking Step Six, it is important to revisit the concept of powerlessness. Instead of telling our Higher Power what it is we want to be—"Make me more motivated," or "Make me more open-minded"—we make a statement of our condition as it is. We state how things are with us: "My Higher Power, I am lazy," or "My Higher Power, I am intolerant of others." Only with this humility will we be ready and willing to have such defects removed.

Even with all the preparation we do for the Sixth Step, we may still have reservations. Even when we know we no longer have any use for our defects of character, we are accustomed to them from years of togetherness. In our minds, our pride and selfishness served us well. We might ask ourselves, "Can I let go of some of my most monumental defects?"

That is why we go to the Seventh Step. It's there that we see our Higher Power doing for us what we really could not do for ourselves. For many, the removal of our shortcomings is the miracle that turns doubters into believers. Step Six is really the "get ready, get set" that builds toward the "go" of Step

Seven—the *action* of asking our Higher Power to remove our shortcomings.

Step Seven: Being Changed

Humbly asked our Higher Power to remove our shortcomings.

The first word in Step Seven is "humbly." Because Step Seven so expressly concerns itself with humility, we need to stop to consider its importance.

Humility is the practice of being humble. It is the recognition of our self-worth and seeing that same God-given worth in other people, even when they are so totally unlike us that we don't understand them or get along with them. Humility is the awareness that we are *not* all-powerful controllers of every aspect of our lives and that we do need the help and guidance of a Higher Power.

"Humbly" asking our Higher Power is quite different from the way we're used to praying—either begging or bargaining. In those cases we prayed to our Higher Power out of desperation. From now on we pray with humility; we humbly ask our Higher Power to remove our shortcomings.

Most people find it easier to ask that their shortcomings be removed gradually or one at a time. Having lived with these shortcomings for so long, it is not so easy to shed them all at once. We need to be patient with ourselves and with our Higher Power during this process. This may take time and a lot of work before we are "entirely ready," as stated in Step Six. We don't expect to become perfect people, but we aim to improve. The goal is progress, not perfection.

We can work this Step alone with our Higher Power, with members of our religious group, in our COPD support groups, or with members of nicotine-cessation support groups—wherever we can trust and be trusted.

And although a personal prayer is our own connection with our Higher Power, when two or three are gathered together, we feel a special bond not only with our Higher Power but also with others who share our condition. We feel this closeness as we say the Serenity Prayer together in our groups.

Our own shortcomings *can,* with our Higher Power's help, be removed.

Step Eight: Preparing for Change

Made a list of all persons we had harmed and became willing to make amends to them all.

In this Step even more strength is added to our program. If there is anybody we have harmed, it is important we get the guilt off our conscience and make a heartfelt attempt to reconcile with them. If we have hurt friends and the friendship has suffered, the benefit is that we might repair that friendship. By making a list, we become clear as to exactly who these people are.

Over the years, our smoking may have caused discomfort to others—to family members, friends, and co-workers. We may have been rude to them when they asked us to stop. Chances are that at the very least we ignored or rebuffed many people's feelings on the subject. Our smoking may have interfered with the family's social relations because friends may not have wanted to come to our home.

We also might want to consider our behavior after we found out we had COPD. It may have been unacceptable. We may have been disrespectful at times to the health professionals who were trying to help us with our recovery. Our COPD probably caused financial hardship to our families, not to mention unspeakable worry. Our list needs to include all persons we have harmed, regardless of how much and under what circumstances.

We may want to put ourselves at the top of our amends list. We are the ones who have suffered the most as a result of our actions. We inhaled into our lungs poisonous substances that caused the life-shortening disease COPD.

Understandably, the prospect of acknowledging our responsibility for hurting others can be daunting. As with the other Steps, this one becomes less frightening once we settle down to do it.

Take your pen or pencil and use the space below to write the names of a few people who make you feel uncomfortable. Don't write why, or anything else. Just put down a list of names.

The simple act of writing down names changes our perspective. Instead of thinking about the harm others have done to us, we take responsibility for the pain we caused in those relationships. It is a profound experience that represents a coming of age.

If you made a list, congratulations. You are halfway through this important Step.

Many of us avoid the Eighth Step because we are already thinking ahead to Step Nine or because we feel too guilty or fearful to face a long list of names. It is important to remember that just because we've written a list does not mean we need to make amends immediately.

The second part of this Step involves willingness. Being willing to make amends means discarding all resentments and accepting responsibility for the harm we have done to others.

In so doing we become completely ready to do whatever we can to make amends for these harms, thereby unburdening ourselves of guilty feelings that interfere with our emotional well-being as we contend with our COPD.

Continuing to Make Amends

This is not a program of perfection. Instead, it stresses progress. Even when we practice the principles of this Twelve Step program in all our affairs, it is inevitable we shall have "run-ins" with other people in our lives (though far fewer than before, it is hoped). For that reason a new and revised Step Eight list is an option for any of us at any time.

Step Nine: Repairing the Past

Made direct amends to such people wherever possible, except when to do so would injure them or others.

We begin making amends to our loved ones by showing them we are caring for ourselves. In addition to giving up smoking, we follow our doctors' recommendations for medication and exercise. No longer do our families and friends have to fear we are trying to kill ourselves. Many of our amends are made by the act of taking appropriate measures to contain our disease.

These, however, are "indirect" amends, and the operative word in Step Nine is "direct." Making amends directly helps us gain humility, honesty, and courage, and that means we need to go directly to the people we have harmed and directly admit our wrongs. Being direct isn't just about righting wrongs; it also inspires us to summon honesty and courage to our service and gives us the freedom to look others in the eye and experience the self-respect we deserve.

Amends need not consist of a lengthy explanation; all that's needed is a heartfelt apology. The person to whom we are making amends may feel some uneasiness too. For this reason, simplicity and directness usually work best when making amends.

Ideally we apologize face-to-face. The very directness of this approach is beneficial. Sometimes this is impractical, however, so we may choose to write a letter, make a phone call, or even, in this electronic age, send an e-mail.

In the vast majority of cases, amends are well received. Even in those rare instances when they are not, this is not a reason to avoid making the effort next time. Almost always, relationships improve markedly when amends are made.

Remember that Steps Eight and Nine also allow us to make amends to *ourselves*. The reward for taking these Steps is a gradual but increasing sense of self-acceptance and self-respect, of being in harmony with our own personal world.

Such feelings are indispensable in our quest to overcome the emotional pain associated with COPD, and experiencing them helps us cope better with the challenges of the disease.

Step Ten: Maintaining My New Life

Continued to take personal inventory and when we were wrong promptly admitted it.

Managing our chronic illness presents us with perhaps the most difficult challenge of our lives. Yet by following the Steps of this program, we have been able to achieve a strong measure of conciliation with ourselves, others, and a Higher Power. To help maintain our serenity, we must try to stay comfortable with ourselves and others. We do this by continuing to take a personal inventory.

We are only human. The path we are taking offers progress, not perfection, so it is inevitable—even with a Higher Power in our lives—that we will do things we know are wrong or misguided. These can be monumental or trivial. Maybe a health setback put into motion thoughts of suicide. Or the expense of a medication caused us to snap angrily at a pharmacist. When defects such as self-pity and anger rear up, we can go back and do a Seventh Step on them, asking our Higher Power to remove these shortcomings.

It helps to get feedback from people close to us—family members, friends, fellow participants of support groups. We need to ask these people to point out our character defects to us if they become apparent.

The second part of this Step emphasizes that if we want to maintain our serenity, we must admit our wrongs "promptly." It is important not to let anything build up inside us that will interfere with our ability to cope with our chronic illness. Once we get used to it, admitting we're wrong can be a liberating sensation that enables us to move on in our lives without unnecessarily harboring resentments or other unhealthy thoughts.

Step Eleven: Partnership with a Higher Power

Sought through prayer and meditation to improve our conscious contact with a Power greater than ourselves, praying only for knowledge of our Higher Power's will and the courage to carry that out.

When coping with a chronic illness like COPD, we need all the help we can get. The help of a Power greater than ourselves is available to us through prayer (talking to our Higher Power) and meditation (listening to our Higher Power). By praying and meditating in our daily lives, we keep a channel open to our Higher Power. We can rely on that Power's strength to help us at any time as we deal with the enormous challenges of our disease.

Step Eleven calls for us to follow our Higher Power's will as it is revealed to us through prayer and meditation. Once we believe we are trying to do our Higher Power's will, we can ask for the strength to carry that out. When we do not feel like exercising or attending a support group meeting, we can ask for encouragement. When we have a compulsion to smoke, we can ask our Higher Power to take it away. Our Higher Power is always with us and is always willing to come to our aid.

It's important for us to remember that although we have turned over the care of our disease to a Higher Power, we need to cooperate with that Power. By attending support groups and listening to others who share our condition, adhering to our doctors' advice, and, above all, *not smoking,* we are doing what is necessary to care for our COPD and ourselves as our Higher Power wishes us to. And in so doing, we will be better able to receive the strength that Power wants to provide.

The Importance of Prayer and Meditation

Medical science has demonstrated that prayer and meditation have a beneficial effect on our health (see page xv). They do this by helping us develop a closer relationship with our Higher Power, an improved "spirit consciousness."

Prayer means talking to our Higher Power. Meditation means listening to our Higher Power. Prayer and meditation don't come easily to everyone. As with most things, the more we do it, the better we get. Those who have cultivated a close relationship with their Higher Power can suggest ways we, too, can do this. We need to seek out such people and consult them or read books on how to meditate.

Perhaps the most often-heard recommendation is to have a quiet time each morning during which we ask our Higher Power for the strength to manage our COPD that day and a similar interlude each night when we thank our Higher Power for helping us to live another day with our chronic illness.

Many people meditate at least thirty minutes a day—a time we may need to work up to. Meditation involves quieting the mind. We can begin meditating by getting in a comfortable position, closing our eyes, and focusing on a word, such as *peace*. At first, many thoughts of what we "should" be doing enter our mind, but we learn to release them. When our minds are quiet, we are able to get in touch with our inner selves and to listen to our Higher Power. Afterward, sometimes miraculously, answers to our problems will just come to us.

The strength we need to cope with our chronic illness comes from communicating with our Higher Power in prayer and meditation. We must actively seek out spirit communication with our Higher Power. This is a matter directly between us and that Power. Those who seek it in formal religious settings do not always receive the full joy and wonder of direct spirit communication. From direct communication comes life, joy, peace, and spiritual healing.

Step Twelve: Carrying the Message

Having had a spiritual awakening as the result of these steps, we tried to carry our message to others with our condition and to practice these principles in all our affairs.

By the time we reach Step Twelve, we've changed. The compulsion to deny our disease and to engage in behaviors that not only caused it but made it worse have been lifted—not by our own power, but by a Power greater than ourselves. This in itself is a spiritual awakening that will help us as we contend with our disease.

If we've worked the Steps, we have the gift of being able to manage our chronic illness. If we haven't worked the program, we now know we have the tools.

Truly one of the best ways to keep this gift is to give it away. We have experience, strength, and hope that we can share with others. We let ourselves be used as a channel for a Higher Power to work through. We can now partake in the joy of helping others to live healthier, happier, and longer lives.

One way we might "give it away" is to make ourselves available as volunteers to those who organize lung disease prevention campaigns. Or we might provide comfort and company to people with COPD living in convalescent homes. If we attend Nicotine Anonymous meetings, we can help make the coffee, set up beforehand, and clean up afterward.

If some member of our support group seems to be dwelling on the negative aspects of his or her life, we might take it upon ourselves to spend some time with this person and try to lend a sympathetic ear and an encouraging word.

Whether you find an organized COPD support group or not, seek out and make friends with two or more other respiratory patients. Make it a point to have breakfast or lunch with them often, phone them regularly, and talk. Praise their efforts, celebrate their successes (no matter how small), and let them do the same for you.

If we practice the principles of this Twelve Step program in all our affairs, we will likely realize our full physical potential with this disease, and an abundance of spirit. We live as our Higher Power intends us to—happy, joyous, and free.

On Spiritual Awakenings

For those unfamiliar with Twelve Step programs, the term *spiritual awakening* can be the subject of confusion. Many people assume that a spiritual awakening is by definition a cataclysmic occurrence—an opening of the heavens accompanied by a chorus of hallelujahs. In the absence of such an event, there is the risk that some of us might assume the program isn't working for us. But instant and dramatic conversions to spirit consciousness are not what the Twelve Steps are predicated on. Although such transformations take place, they are by no means the rule. Most spiritual awakenings are simple—very simple—yet the feeling we leave with is profound. We feel enlightened and in awe.

A spiritual awakening could be as simple as a thought we have while walking through the woods or watching a child. It could be suddenly seeing ourselves or others in a totally different light. It could be running into someone who gives us the answer to the question we've been asking ourselves.

A person may have one big spiritual awakening, but most people have many smaller-scale awakenings. As the Twelve Steps become our guide to living well with COPD and as we develop a relationship with a Power greater than ourselves who loves us and cares for us, we come to an understanding of what is truly meant by the words *spiritual awakening.*

Step by Step

We're now aware of the Twelve Steps and what they mean. They aren't always easy to accept or understand, because the program, as we have heard, is *simple* but not *easy.* We pause on landings along the way: after the first three Steps (acceptance, hope, faith), after Steps Four through Seven (inner housecleaning), again after Eight and Nine (relationships with other people), and finally after the summing-up (Steps Ten, Eleven, and Twelve).

We make some important discoveries about our inner selves, about how we relate to others, and about our spiritual links to a Higher Power. As we go back over these Steps again and again, understanding them a little better each time, they begin to feel more solid under our feet.

We learn to transcend the emotional pain of our chronic illness and to take measures that will help our condition. In spite of overwhelming odds, we're happy—most of the time—we're interested in life, and we're growing.

These are our own personal miracles, for which we are endlessly grateful.

CHAPTER THREE

Medical Guidelines
for Containing COPD

By practicing the principles of a Twelve Step program in your daily affairs, you will come to experience the serenity you need to live the rest of your life with COPD. Above all, you will have learned to "turn over" your disease to the care of a Higher Power. You are now working with that Power.

Serenity doesn't mean apathy. Part of your responsibility to your Higher Power is to do all that is necessary to care for yourself. It might help if you adopt the assertive attitude of a Bill Horden, a lay expert on COPD (who describes himself not as a patient advocate, but an *im*patient advocate).[1] "COPD isn't a death sentence," Bill states unequivocally. "It isn't untreatable, it isn't necessarily progressive, it

---

1. If you are interested in becoming an advocate for federal action on behalf of COPD patients, contact the Coalititon for Pulmonary Patient Care, a grassroots coalition of patients and families of patients who suffer with COPD. Their Internet address is http://members.xoom.com/CPPC_USA

isn't necessarily crippling, and it isn't a single disease, so it never affects two people in exactly the same way."

Bill Horden's approach to managing his own COPD has enabled him to actually improve his quality of life. "I'm now sixty-eight years old, and I've felt better, been more active, eaten better, and been happier the last two years than at any time during the preceding three or four," he says.

People like Bill Horden benefit by taking a proactive attitude toward their disease. Being proactive means getting qualified medical care, enrolling in a multidisciplinary rehabilitation/wellness program, and joining or even forming a support group composed of other men and women with COPD.

Medical Care

You require the services of respiratory care specialists who will provide you with the aggressive treatment you need, since family physicians are usually not as qualified to treat this disease. The concern is that general practitioners will prescribe rote treatment regimens that do not take into consideration the unique character of each person's COPD and his or her ability to cope with it.

Your family doctor should be able to refer you to a

top-of-the-line respiratory care specialist. The names of prominent respiratory care specialists can also be found in the listings of pulmonary rehabilitation/wellness centers in the appendix.

A Rehabilitation/Wellness Program

If you have been diagnosed with COPD, particularly a moderate to severe form of it, you will benefit enormously from a pulmonary rehabilitation/wellness program. The purpose of such programs is to teach you how to manage your disease, both medically and emotionally.

Try to get into a program that is multidisciplinary, employing the services of pulmonologists, respiratory therapists, physical therapists, pharmacologists, dietitians, occupational therapists, and psychologists. The most successful programs last six to eight weeks. If no such program exists in your area, or if your insurance doesn't cover such a program, by all means enroll in one of the less intensive rehabilitation programs that are offered at the closest location to you. But be assertive. Encourage the people running that program to make it as comprehensive and challenging as possible for you and the other participants.

Refer to the appendix for listings of pulmonary rehabilitation/wellness centers.

Support Groups

After you complete your wellness program, make every effort to participate in a COPD support group, even if you don't believe it's for you. The relief that comes from sharing thoughts, feelings, and coping strategies with people who are in the same position as you can be monumental. Don't discount the importance of these groups before you've given them a fair chance. Attend at least six meetings with an open mind before you decide whether they're for you.

The American Lung Association sponsors "Better Breathing Clubs" in most major cities. These are support groups specifically for people with lung disorders.[2] Many hospitals host support groups for people with chronic illnesses such as COPD. Check with your doctor for groups in your area.

A support group should meet at least once or twice a week for one or two hours at a time. Although some people recommend that a therapist be present to guide the discussion in a COPD support group, many groups (including Twelve Step programs like Nicotine Anonymous) offer excellent support for their members without the services of paid professionals.

The role of a therapist in a COPD support group is,

2. For information on a Better Breathing Club near you, contact the American Lung Association National Headquarters at 1740 Broadway, New York, NY 10019, (212) 315-8700.

in part, to make sure that the discussion does not focus on the negative. In a group without a therapist present, participants must remember that while a support group is a place to share hardships, the emphasis is on the positive progress the participants have made since starting therapy. Certain meetings should also be set aside for spouses and family members to attend.

Maybe there are no support groups in your area, in which case you can think about starting one yourself. Get advice about starting a group from one of the health professionals on staff or call an existing group in another location.

You may decide to use the Twelve Steps as the basis for the support group you form. Why not? After all, the Steps have been used with extraordinary success by people dealing with a variety of other chronic illnesses. If you do decide to make yours a Twelve Step group, learn how to run it by talking to the Alcoholics Anonymous World Services office in New York or to someone who is very familiar with Twelve Step groups. A longtime member of Alcoholics Anonymous, Nicotine Anonymous, Overeaters Anonymous, or Al-Anon (a Twelve Step program for family members and adult children of alcoholics) would be ideal. That person might recommend that you also incorporate the Twelve Traditions of AA as guidelines for how to organize your group.

If it isn't practical for you to attend or start a support group (perhaps because of your geographical location or the advanced stage of your COPD), or even if you *are* a regular participant in such a group, consider getting involved in an Internet "chat room" for people with COPD. One of the best-organized of these forums can be found on the Colorado HealthNet Internet site (www.coloradohealthnet.org). Simply called the COPD Forum, it has regular participants who were diagnosed with COPD a long time ago and thus can share helpful coping strategies with those who are newly diagnosed.

Colorado HealthNet, a nonprofit organization, also has an innovative "Pen Pals" program wherein people with chronic illnesses, their caregivers, families, and friends can find people with similar problems to share ideas, coping strategies, hopes, knowledge, and friendship. Pen Pals is a place for you to communicate one-on-one by e-mail with another person whom you have found compatible.

Through a support group and by communicating and interacting with others who share your disease, you may discover that having COPD has presented you with the opportunity to address issues that would otherwise have remained unmanaged and which, having been dealt with, will make you a more complete person.

What Is a Support Group?

Support groups consist of people who have come together to share the common experiences and problems unique to their disease or condition. In addition to being a place to meet people who share a common bond, self-help/ support groups also help members in other ways. Through newsletters and regular contact with other people in similar situations, members receive up-to-date information regarding their disability and the treatments that are available. Along with this sharing comes understanding and a sense of belonging. Research confirms that the coming together of people in trouble serves to increase self-esteem, decrease anxiety and depression, and raise levels of overall well-being.

Information on support groups in your area can be found in a variety of ways. Local newspapers often offer feature listings. Handbooks of community resources, including support groups, are usually available in local libraries and hospitals. Particularly active groups are often listed in the Yellow Pages under "Social Service Agencies." Major national groups such as the American Lung Association can provide you with information about support groups in your area.

Complementing these three pillars of COPD management are several important medical components of a program to contain your COPD. They include behavior modification, infection prevention/early intervention, medication, oxygen therapy, environment awareness, and breathlessness controls.

Feel Better? Watch Out!

If you follow the guidelines in this book, you will soon start to feel better. Do not take this as permission to cut back on the efforts you are making; it is not time to think about picking up a cigarette, skipping an exercise session or a support group meeting, eating poorly, or neglecting your medications. Remember what made you feel better in the first place!

Behavior Modification

If you haven't done these already, it's vital for you to make several important lifestyle changes if you want to improve your condition.

Stop Smoking

Right now the most important action you must take is to stop smoking—or, if you've already quit, to make every effort to stay quit. Unless you stop smoking you will perpetuate the long-term damage to your lungs that caused your COPD. In the short term, smoking will irritate the air passages in your lungs, causing them to generate excess phlegm, which in turn provides a fertile breeding ground for infections.

A variety of options are available for people who want to stop smoking. Dozens of inpatient and outpatient smoking cessation programs exist around the country. Your doctor may be able to refer you to a program.

Nicotine replacement therapy may also play a useful role in smoking cessation. Forms of nicotine replacement include gum, the patch, the inhaler, and pills. Research shows that these products work best when combined with some form of behavior therapy. Just as the Twelve Steps are the foundation of recovery from mood-altering drugs such as nicotine and alcohol, nicotine replacement products can serve as essential tools for quitting smoking. Read up on the differences between the nicotine replacement therapies and talk to your physician about whether they are an advisable option for you.

The Twelve Steps can also serve as key tools for quitting smoking. Nicotine Anonymous (NA), a Twelve Step mutual-help support group, can be the starting point for smokers trying to quit or can serve as continuing care for people who complete an inpatient or outpatient smoking cessation program. If there is no listing for Nicotine Anonymous in your local telephone book, check the organization's detailed Internet site for the meeting that is convenient to where you live or work (www.nicotine-anonymous.org).

The Health Benefits of Quitting Smoking

Quitting smoking has immediate and significant benefits.

Your circulation quickly improves, and the deadly carbon monoxide levels in your blood start to decline. Your heart rate and blood pressure, which are unhealthily elevated by smoking, go down. Your senses of taste and smell come back within days, and breathing gets steadily easier.

In the long term, people who stop smoking live longer than those who continue with their cigarette habit. After ten to fifteen years, an ex-smoker's risk of an early death is approximately that of a person who has never smoked.

Stopping smoking dramatically lowers your chance of getting cancer, and this risk continues to decline the longer you stay "smoke-free." Lung cancer is the leading cause of cancer death, and the main risk factor for lung cancer is smoking cigarettes. After a person quits smoking, the risk of developing lung cancer gradually declines until, within ten years, the risk is 30 to 50 percent below that of a person who continues to smoke. The risk of contracting cancers of the mouth, throat, and esophagus lessens significantly by five years after quitting.

Smoking cessation will benefit you whatever your age. Some older men and women claim they don't feel the benefits of quitting. However, research shows that people sixty to sixty-four years old who quit smoking are 10 percent less likely to die during the next fifteen years than their peers who continue to smoke. Those who quit before age fifty experience even greater health rewards, and their risk of dying in the next fifteen years is half that of smokers.

Exercise

Exercise is a lifestyle "must" for everyone, but it has special implications if you have COPD. Why? Because exercise makes your lungs more efficient as they adapt to increased demands. That means your lungs are better able to respond to the requirements of daily activities.

Unfortunately, though, a vicious cycle of inactivity often develops if you have COPD. You may generally feel breathless at lower levels of activity than a person with healthy lungs. To avoid this sensation, you reduce your level of activity, which leads to greater deconditioning, which in turn increases breathlessness at even lower levels of activity. The cycle continues until even the most benign daily activities—eating, for example—cause disabling shortages of breath.

The following are some general guidelines for safe and successful exercise participation by people with COPD:

- Doc talk: If you have COPD, it is absolutely essential that you speak with your doctor before starting an exercise program.
- Ease on in: Start off at a pace you can easily sustain; then increase the intensity of your program as you go on.
- Goal orientation: Set realistic but challenging goals for your exercise program. If you choose walking as your main form of exercise, increase the intensity of your walking program by following the table shown on pages 63–65. Your ultimate goal is to work up to at least three moderate exercise sessions per week that each last between forty and seventy minutes.
- Decisions, decisions: Choose the right activity. Depending on the severity of your condition, certain sports may be beyond your capabilities. Walking is an excellent form of exercise for

people with COPD, and it can be done as a group social activity. You could even propose to make walking part of your support group program.

- Buddy up: If it's not practical for you to get your entire support group exercising together, try at least to find a friend or two who will exercise with you. That way you'll motivate each other, and you'll find yourself less likely to cancel a workout for fear of letting someone else down.

- Whose workout is it, anyway?: Though it helps to get motivated by exercising with others, remember to set your own pace. You aren't competing against anyone but yourself. Let your exercise partners know how you feel.

- Danger signs: If you become nauseated or dizzy, weak, short of breath, have palpitations, or experience pain, stop exercising immediately. You may want to consult your doctor, depending on the degree of pain or discomfort.

- Cool it: Take time to cool down after your workout. Slow down toward the end of your activity; then stretch for a few minutes after you stop.

- Here's to you: When you achieve a goal—however modest—take time to congratulate yourself. Consider giving yourself a small reward. You deserve it!

A Walking Program for People with COPD

The walking program described here is designed for people with mild to moderate COPD. Even if you have severe COPD, you can do the walking sessions described in the early part of the program. Each walking session is divided into three parts—the warm-up phase, the target zone phase, and the cool-down phase. Of these three phases, the target zone requires explanation.

Achieving the Target Zone
To get the maximum benefit from exercise, it is necessary to exercise hard enough that your heart and lungs are working at between 60 and 75 percent of their maximum capabilities.

To check to see if you're exercising within your target zone, you need to take your pulse while you're exercising. Here's how:

- *Place the tips of your fingers over one of the major blood vessels (try just to the left or right of your Adam's apple or the spot on the inside of your wrist below the bone of your thumb).*
- *Count the number of times your heart beats during a ten-second period. Then multiply that number by six to figure out how many times a minute your heart is beating.*
- *Compare your heart rate with the chart on the following page. For instance, if you are sixty-*

*five years old, your goal is to have a target
zone of between 78 and 116 beats per minute
(as someone with COPD, you can expect to be
in the high range of that variance).*

Age	Target Heart Rate Zone
20 years	100–150 beats per minute
25 years	98–146 beats per minute
30 years	95–142 beats per minute
35 years	93–138 beats per minute
40 years	90–135 beats per minute
45 years	88–131 beats per minute
50 years	85–127 beats per minute
55 years	83–123 beats per minute
60 years	80–120 beats per minute
65 years	78–116 beats per minute
70 years	75–113 beats per minute

	Warm-Up Phase	Target Zone Phase	Cool-Down Phase	Total
Week 1				
Session A	Walk normally, 5 min.	Walk fast, 5 min.	Walk normally, 5 min.	15 min.
Session B	repeat	repeat	repeat	15 min.
Session C	repeat	repeat	repeat	15 min.

Each week do the walking session three times, as shown for week one. If you find you reach a point where the sessions leave you overly fatigued (tired enough that you don't think you could go to the next level), repeat that week's program until you think you are fit enough to move on to the next level. It isn't necessary for you to complete the program in twelve weeks.

	Warm-Up Phase	Target Zone Phase	Cool-Down Phase	Total
Week 2	Walk normally, 5 min.	Walk fast, 7 min.	Walk normally, 5 min.	17 min.
Week 3	Walk normally, 5 min.	Walk fast, 9 min.	Walk normally, 5 min.	19 min.
Week 4	Walk normally, 5 min.	Walk fast, 11 min.	Walk normally, 5 min.	21 min.
Week 5	Walk normally, 5 min.	Walk fast, 13 min.	Walk normally, 5 min.	23 min.
Week 6	Walk normally, 5 min.	Walk fast, 15 min.	Walk normally, 5 min.	25 min.
Week 7	Walk normally, 5 min.	Walk fast, 18 min.	Walk normally, 5 min.	28 min.

	Warm-Up Phase	Target Zone Phase	Cool-Down Phase	Total
Week 8	Walk normally, 5 min.	Walk fast, 20 min.	Walk normally, 5 min.	30 min.
Week 9	Walk normally, 5 min.	Walk fast, 23 min.	Walk normally, 5 min.	33 min.
Week 10	Walk normally, 5 min.	Walk fast, 26 min.	Walk normally, 5 min.	36 min.
Week 11	Walk normally, 5 min.	Walk fast, 28 min.	Walk normally, 5 min.	38 min.
Week 12	Walk normally, 5 min.	Walk fast, 30 min.	Walk normally, 5 min.	40 min.

Week 13 onwards: Remember to check your pulse periodically during the target zone phase to make sure you are exercising in that zone. As your lungs adapt to the demands of this walking program, try exercising in the upper range of your target zone. Gradually increase your fast-walking time to between thirty and sixty minutes three or four times a week. With a five-minute warm-up and cool-down period, your walking sessions should last forty to seventy minutes.

Improve Your Diet

There is no special diet for a person with COPD. Good nutrition, though, can improve your energy level, lung function, exercise tolerance, and weight and can also prevent your chance of getting a cold or a flu, all of which are very important for someone with a chronic illness.

The following nutrition tips are from the American Association for Respiratory Care.[3] However, they are guidelines only. If you have any concerns about your diet, consult your physician or a registered dietitian/nutritionist.

1. Eat foods daily from each of the basic food groups: fruits and vegetables, dairy products, cereal and grains, and protein.
2. Limit your salt intake. Too much sodium can cause you to retain fluids that may interfere with breathing.
3. Limit your intake of caffeinated drinks. Caffeine may interfere with some of your medications and may also make you feel nervous.
4. Avoid foods that produce gas or make you feel bloated, which could increase your discomfort. The best process to use in eliminating foods from your diet is trial and error.

3. These guidelines are used with the permission of the American Association for Respiratory Care (AARC), 11030 Ables Lane, Dallas, TX 75224, (972) 243-2272.

5. Try to eat your main meal early. This way, you will have lots of energy to carry you through the day.

6. Choose foods that are easy to prepare. Don't waste all of your energy preparing a meal. Try to rest before eating so that you can enjoy your meal.

7. Avoid foods that supply little or no nutritional value. An unhealthy diet will only make you feel worse.

8. Try eating six small meals a day instead of three large ones. This will keep you from filling up your stomach and causing shortness of breath.

9. If you are using oxygen, be sure to wear your cannula while eating and after meals too. Eating and digestion require energy, which causes your body to use more oxygen.

10. Try to eat in a relaxed atmosphere. It takes a lot of effort for someone with COPD to eat, and eating when under stress adds extra difficulty. To get the most from your meals, make them attractive and enjoyable.

11. Consult your physician if you have other dietary restrictions, such as ulcers, or if you are overweight or underweight.

12. In many states, there are agencies that will

provide meals for people for a small fee or at no charge. Check with local church organizations or government agencies to see what is available in your area.

A proper diet will not cure your disease, but it will make you feel better. Good nutrition and a balanced diet are essential to everyone's health; but because you have lung disease, you must be even more careful than most about following good nutrition guidelines.

Manage Your Stress

For most people, increased stress is an inevitable consequence of chronic illness. Tension, however, can cause shortness of breath, not to mention poorer quality of mental health.

One of the most effective ways to deal with stress is prayer. Praying evokes beneficial changes in the human body, such as decreases in blood pressure, heart rates, and breathing, all of which are characteristics of the "relaxation response." The relaxation response produces a spiritual feeling in about 25 percent of people—even the nonreligious, according to Herbert Benson, the Harvard Medical School doctor who first described the effect. Several studies have indicated that having others pray for you also has a positive effect on healing.

What is particularly effective is a short invocation

that can be said at any time you feel stress. It is known as the "Serenity Prayer."

> God, grant me the serenity
> To accept the things I cannot change,
> The courage to change the things I can,
> And the wisdom to know the difference.

These are some other ways to deal with stress:

- Exercise.
- Take time to relax with a good book, movie, or music.
- Develop new interests, or rekindle interests in past activities (e.g., take a course).
- Interact with family and friends.
- Address a person or situation that's causing you stress.
- Join a support group.
- Try meditation, yoga, massage, or acupuncture/acupressure.
- Learn about your disease, but don't obsess about it.

Yoga for COPD

Yoga is an ancient system of exercises practiced as part of a discipline to promote control of the body and mind. Experts say yoga offers specific exercises and techniques you can do yourself to help with a variety of ailments.

The following yoga exercises can help people with COPD learn to breathe more efficiently:

- *Place your fingertips on your shoulders. Breathe in and bring your elbows together so they meet in front of your chest. Lift your elbows as high as you can; then exhale as you trace five circles with your elbows.*
- *Sit on a stool. Make a breaststroke motion with your arms, slowly stretching them behind you. Clasp your hands, lowering your arms below your buttocks, and pull your shoulders back. Then, still clasping your hands behind you, breathe in and lift your arms up as far as you can. Breathe out, lower your arms, and unclasp your hands.*

Repeat ten times or as much as you can tolerate and do each exercise three or four times a day.

Infection Prevention/Early Intervention

When you have COPD, infections in your lungs are dangerous. They can make you very ill very quickly. A lung infection is a likely reason you may have to be hospitalized. The most common and dangerous kind of infection you need to beware of if you have COPD is influenza, or "the flu."

Get a Flu Vaccination

If you have COPD, you are at high risk of getting the flu. And people with COPD who come down with the flu get sicker and their condition lasts longer than those with healthy lungs. It is essential if you have COPD that you get a flu vaccination every year. Vaccinations are done annually in October and November at your health clinic for a nominal fee.

Other Ways to Prevent Infection

In addition to getting an annual flu shot, talk to your doctor about getting a onetime pneumonia vaccination. Also, wash your hands frequently and avoid large crowds in poorly ventilated places. Smoking increases your chances of developing an infection, so again, it is crucial that you quit smoking.

If You Get an Infection

If you have COPD, your lungs have lost much of their natural defenses. Therefore, an infection is a real problem because you'll get sicker and the infection will last longer than if you had normal resistance. Because even a mild infection needs to be treated right away, you must be alert to any signs that you may be getting an infection.

Here are some of the signs:

- You're coughing up an unusually large amount of phlegm.
- Your phlegm has changed color to yellow, brown, or green.
- You have seen blood in your phlegm.
- You feel more out of breath than usual.
- You have a fever.
- You feel in poor health, have no stamina, and lack energy.

Those who have acute and severe lung infections may act confused and disorientated, and their speech may be slurred. This is because their blocked airways are unable to deliver enough oxygen to their brains.

Antibiotics are the most important component of medical treatment for bacterial lung infections of the kind commonly suffered by people with COPD. However, contrary to many people's misconceptions, antibiotics are ineffective against viral infections such as the flu and the common cold, and you should not insist your doctor prescribe you with antibiotics for these conditions. For more information on the proper use of antibiotics to treat lung infections, see below.

Some Advice about Antibiotics

Antibiotics are your first line of defense against lung infections. Certain precautions should be observed, however, whenever taking antibiotics.

- *Listen carefully to your doctor's directions on how to take your prescription—how often, for how long, whether with or without meals. Read the prescription carefully.*
- *To avoid negative interactions, make sure the prescribing doctor is aware of all other medications you are taking.*
- *Don't discontinue taking your medications—even if you start feeling better. If you don't finish taking all the medication, you may kill only some of the bacteria. The remaining bacteria may get stronger, making your next infection more resistant to antibiotics.*
- *Don't take an antibiotic left over from a previous illness or ones prescribed for someone else.*
- *Report unexpected side effects such as rashes or stomach upsets so your doctor can prescribe a different antibiotic or a change in dosage or schedule.*

Medications for COPD

Medication is a cornerstone of COPD containment.

The drugs described in this section are those medications that address the basic problem associated with COPD: airway obstruction. Certainly you may be taking other drugs, such as flu vaccines (page 71) or antibiotics for infection (page 72), but these are not used to open up the airways.

Medications for opening up the airways are classified depending on the two ways they work: *bronchodilation* and *anti-inflammatory.*

Bronchodilators are medicines that open up your airways. They are prescribed in pill, liquid, or inhalant form. There are two main types of bronchodilators—beta-agonists and anticholinergics. Beta-agonists work by relaxing the muscles around the airways, while anticholinergics stop the airways from contracting. Often the most effective form of bronchodilator therapy is a combination of both beta-agonists and anticholinergics; this simultaneously relaxes the muscles around the airways and opens the airways up. Bronchodilators are associated with several unpleasant side effects, including muscle tremor, increases in blood pressure and heart rate, restlessness, anxiety, and headaches.

Anti-inflammatories decrease the inflammation inside the airways. Such inflammation includes fluid and cellular debris that tend to clog the airways of people with COPD. Steroids, sometimes called *corticosteroids,* are one type of anti-inflammatory drug. They usually work best in people with COPD who also have asthma. However, there are some COPD-only sufferers who do respond well to corticosteroids. If your airway obstruction cannot be kept under control with bronchodilators, your doctor may initiate a short trial to determine if you respond well to steroids. A typical trial lasts two to three weeks.

Corticosteroids do not have immediate effects and must be used on an ongoing basis to be useful. They are of no value when results are needed in minutes.

Patients usually start steroid therapy by taking steroid pills. Corticosteroid pills are used when inflammation becomes severe. These pills (sometimes known as prednisone) reduce inflammation, swelling, and mucus and help bronchodilators work better. The pills start to work within a few hours but may take several days to take full effect. Although corticosteroid pills may be extremely effective in getting the inflammation under control, they are usually used for only short periods of time, since there are many side effects if used long term, such as water retention, bruising, puffy face, increased appetite, weight gain, and stomach irritation.

In addition, long-term use of oral corticosteroids curbs the body's natural production of corticosteroids. Treatment lasting more than a few weeks may be gradually withdrawn to give the body time to readjust. Some people, however, do well on low doses of oral prednisone for years at a time.

Many patients can eventually switch from the pills to low-dosage inhalers. At low doses, corticosteroid inhalers have few side effects. At moderate and high doses, side effects include hoarseness, sore throat, and, more significantly, thrush, or yeast infection in the mouth and throat. Throat infections can, however, be prevented by rinsing the mouth and gargling and by using what's called a *spacer* (a small holding chamber that attaches to the inhaler).

No two people with lung disease are the same. You need to work with your doctor to establish which medications are best for you—and in what dosages. You will probably have to try several types of medications in different combinations before you hit upon the medication therapy that suits you best. What's important is that you work closely with your doctor and pharmacist to get the most out of the medications currently available on the market.

If you have more than one doctor, make sure each one knows the medicines you are currently taking and for what reasons. Always be sure to ask what your medications are for. Report positive and negative effects. Tell your doctor if any medicine is too expensive for you to keep buying. There may be a cheaper alternative. And if you have any questions, do not hesitate to ask. If you are unsure about the recommendations you are getting, seek a second and third opinion.

Oxygen Therapy

Oxygen therapy benefits people with advanced COPD who have very low oxygen levels. Technological advances have made portable oxygen therapy a viable option for such people. Previously such therapy would have been available only in a hospital setting. Oxygen therapy reduces the symptoms of advanced COPD and in doing so improves physical and mental energy. Symptoms at this stage may include severe shortness of breath, heart strain, headaches, sleeplessness, muscle-wasting, high blood pressure, and, in men, impotence. Many more people than ever before are using portable oxygen, enabling them to live active, productive lives.

Your insurance policy may pay for all your oxygen, but reimbursement will be based on lab results, diagnosis, and other information. Your oxygen equipment and services provider may be able to answer your questions about coverage.

To receive oxygen therapy you will need a prescription from a doctor. The prescription will provide details including how much oxygen you need in liters per minute (LPM), which is calculated based on a blood test you take to measure the oxygen level in your blood (an accurate measure of how well or poorly your lungs are working). It will also say when you need to use the oxygen. Needs vary greatly—some people with COPD use oxygen all the time, while others use it only when sleeping or exercising.

Oxygen comes in small tanks or units you can carry. From these systems there are three different ways of delivering the oxygen to the user. A *nasal cannula* is a two-pronged device that inserts into the nostrils and is kept in place by tubing that rests on the ears or attaches to eyeglass frames. A *mask* is more suitable if you need a high flow of oxygen. Some people alternate between a cannula and mask—using the cannula under normal circumstances and the mask when they need a higher oxygen intake, such as at night or when they have a cold. *Transtracheal* oxygen therapy involves the permanent insertion of a catheter into the windpipe (trachea). The catheter is held in place by a necklace-like device that hangs around the neck. If oxygen flow is more than four LPM, a humidifying component is added to the catheter to prevent excessive dryness.

Safety

Carefully follow the safety guidelines provided by the home medical equipment and services company that provides the equipment. Although oxygen does not burn, it helps other things burn faster, so you need to be particularly aware of inflammation hazards.

- Do not allow anyone to smoke in the room where you are using oxygen (secondhand smoke should be avoided anyway). Put up no-smoking signs in your home. *Never smoke while using oxygen!*
- If you are going to be using oxygen at a restaurant, ask to be seated in the no-smoking section.

- Indoors, make sure the tank is at least ten feet away from any open flame, gas stoves, pilot lights in water heaters and furnaces, and wood-burning stoves.
- Also keep it ten feet away from any electrical equipment that might spark.

In addition, if you use an oxygen concentrator, notify your electric company that you will need priority service if there is a power failure. And do not set the flow rate higher than that prescribed by your doctor, as a flow rate that is too high can damage your lungs and may even make breathing more difficult.

Avoiding Environmental Hazards

There are numerous unseen threats to the lungs of a person who has COPD. These include air pollution, secondhand smoke, strong odors and fumes, and significant temperature changes. If you have COPD, your lungs are not able to defend themselves against these hazards like the lungs of a person who does not have this disease. As a result, you are more susceptible to lung damage, lung infections, and attacks of breathlessness caused by environmental hazards.

The following are some steps you can take to prevent your COPD symptoms from worsening as a result of hazards in the environment.

Air Pollution

Dirt and fumes from air pollution build up in your lungs and can cause lung damage, lung infections, and attacks of breathlessness. In addition, gasses such as carbon monoxide are poisonous and deprive your blood of oxygen. Avoid situations where you might be exposed to polluted air, such as traffic jams, enclosed parking garages, and dusty work areas. During smoggy periods, check television and radio reports for air pollution alerts. When air pollution is heavy, stay indoors with the windows closed and use air-conditioning. Consider using an air filter or air purifier. Avoid housecleaning that raises dust levels in the air.

Secondhand Smoke

Smoke from other people's cigarettes, cigars, or pipes has the same effect as air pollution—it can damage your lungs, cause lung infections, and provoke attacks of breathlessness. Ask smokers to respect your need for clean air. Put up no-smoking signs at home. Avoid smoke-filled rooms. At restaurants, ask to be seated in the no-smoking section.

Strong Odors and Fumes

Microscopic airborne debris from numerous products such as cleaners, paints, glues, and aerosol sprays can damage your lungs, cause lung infections, and provoke attacks of breathlessness. Avoid such products. Don't wear perfumes and ask those close to you to do the same. Avoid toiletries that are excessively scented. When cooking, turn on your kitchen fan, which should be vented outdoors.

Temperature Changes

Cold air can put extra stress on your lungs and can lead to attacks of breathlessness. Breathing through your nose instead of your mouth helps warm the air before it gets to your lungs. Stay indoors during cold weather. If you cannot avoid going outside, cover your nose and mouth with a scarf. Cold-weather masks are available in many pharmacies. If you live 3,500 feet above sea level, relocating to a lower altitude will help you breathe easier. Humid weather may also make you feel worse and can also worsen the effects of air pollution in a person with COPD. In excessively humid weather, stay indoors in an area that is air-conditioned and/or dehumidified.

Learning to Control Breathlessness: "SOS for SOB"

Acute attacks of breathlessness are a way of life for most people with COPD. The feelings of panic associated with these episodes can be terrifying, not to mention physically draining and potentially life-threatening due to the risk of heart failure.

Preventing an acute attack of breathlessness is key, and you have learned several ways to do this in this chapter. It is also important to know what to do when such an episode cannot be avoided. This knowledge allows you to remain calm and prevent the situation from worsening.

When an attack of breathlessness occurs, two simple breathing techniques will help you release the trapped stale air in your lungs and inhale more fresh air.

Pursed-Lip Breathing

- Breathe in slowly through your nose until your lungs feel full.
- Purse your lips as if to whistle.
- Exhale slowly through your pursed lips, taking twice as long to let the air out as you did to breathe it in. Don't force it—let the air escape naturally.
- Do pursed-lip breathing until you are no longer short of breath.

Diaphragmatic Breathing

- Relax your shoulders, put one hand on your abdomen, the other on your chest, and then make your abdomen push out while you breathe in through your nose (although the hand on your abdomen should move, the hand on your chest should not).

- Breathe out slowly through pursed lips. Your abdomen should return to its normal shape.
- Do diaphragmatic breathing until you are no longer short of breath.

As soon as these breathing techniques become second nature, you will be able to use them to alleviate attacks of breathlessness wherever you are. Pursed-lip breathing and diaphragmatic breathing are more effective when combined with appropriate posture—whether you are sitting or standing.

1. Sitting

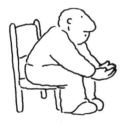

Sit in a chair with your head and shoulders rolled forward and slightly downward (an exaggerated "slouch"). Relax. Rest your forearms on your thighs, palms turned upward. Don't lean on your hands. Keep your feet on the floor and turn your knees outward slightly. Do either pursed-lip breathing or diaphragmatic breathing until you are no longer short of breath.

2. Sitting or standing

Place a pillow on a table. Sit on a chair facing the table, fold your arms, and rest them on the pillow. Lean forward and rest 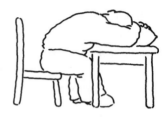 your head sideways on your arms (face either left or right). Do either pursed-lip breathing or diaphragmatic breathing until you are no longer short of breath.

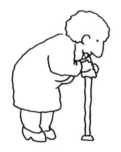

You can also do this position while standing—rest your head on your arms on a countertop, the back of a chair, or other elevated surfaces of an appropriate height.

3. Standing

Lean with your back against a solid surface such as a wall, pole, or pillar. Keep your feet slightly apart, your head and shoulders relaxed. Do either pursed-lip breathing or diaphragmatic breathing until you are no longer short of breath.

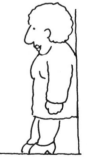

Remember that if you have a chronic illness, you need emotional and psychological healing as well as medical treatment. Such healing is available from several sources. Developing spiritual strength helps people persevere, and even thrive, in the face of the most overwhelming odds, including a life-threatening disease. A Twelve Step program is one way you might develop spiritual strength. You might also consider joining a religious group, or if you are a member of such a group, you might re-examine the quality of your faith. And never forget that the straightforward but profound act of reaching out to help others—even though you yourself might be very ill—will fortify you and strengthen your spirituality.

CHAPTER FOUR

Twenty-Four Hours a Day with COPD[1]

Learning to live with your disease one day at a time is the most effective way to cope with the emotional pain of COPD. By working the Twelve Step spiritual program, you maintain an ongoing relationship with a Higher Power, perform daily inventories and make amends regularly, pray and meditate daily, and share your struggles as often as possible with other nicotine addicts and COPD sufferers.

Nevertheless, a spiritual program works best when supported by practical knowledge. If you treat your self-care as a series of rituals, however, attending to the practicalities can also be a spiritual experience.

The following hints and suggestions were created by members of the Respiratory Club, a support group for pulmonary patients and their families jointly sponsored

1. Parts of this chapter are reprinted with permission from *Round the Clock with COPD,* copyright 1996 by the American Lung Association.

by the American Lung Association of Connecticut and Gaylord Hospital in Wallingford, Connecticut.

In keeping with the belief that chronic illnesses are best coped with by addressing them day to day, the information chronologically follows the schedule people would observe throughout the day.

Pacing

Pacing, or regulating the tempo of daily living, is one of the most important disciplines you will have to learn. Being aware that your limits fluctuate from day to day, even from hour to hour, will help you determine the appropriate pace.

Some mornings you will wake up and know almost immediately it is a day for just relaxing. Or you may awake feeling wonderful and up to a special task you have been saving for a good day. The important thing is to learn to trust your own feelings and to go with them. Don't take on more than you can handle comfortably. When you feel tired, quit.

There will, of course, be many occasions when you may want to expend a little more physical energy than usual. These could range from washing windows to enjoying sex.

It is healthy for you to exert yourself if you do it with a little common sense. Here are a few suggestions:

1. Wait until an hour or more after eating. Digestion draws blood, which contains oxygen, away from muscles, leaving them less able to cope with extra demands.
2. You may find you feel your best soon after taking your medicine (so long as you don't take it right after eating).
3. If you have an inhaler, use it before performing tasks that require special effort, being careful never to inhale more than prescribed.
4. Pace yourself and don't rush.
5. If you feel breathless, use pursed-lip breathing or diaphragmatic breathing techniques (see pages 82–83). Remember, they really help, and you can do them anytime, anyplace.

Sexuality and COPD

For people with COPD, attacks of acute breathlessness are a common occurrence during sexual activity. Often these symptoms are triggered by the stress associated with the fear of such an attack, and not the exertion of sex itself. As a result, many men and women with COPD avoid sexual intimacy altogether. Their partners may also believe that sex should be avoided too, lest it trigger a dangerous episode of acute breathlessness.

However, staying sexually active is important for people with chronic illnesses. It helps maintain a sense of connection with significant others and reinforces self-esteem.

The following are some guidelines to help you enjoy a fulfilling sex life while living with COPD:

- *Use a bronchodilator before—and, if necessary, during—sex.*
- *Cough up phlegm before sex.*
- *Ask your partner not to apply heavily scented products to his or her hair or body that might trigger a lung reaction in you (perfumes, hair sprays, etc.).*
- *Ask your partner to take a more active role.*
- *Choose positions that are less demanding.*
- *Choose a comfortable environment, paying special attention to room temperature so you don't get too hot (the anxiety associated with heat can trigger episodes of breathlessness).*
- *Avoid having sex after eating a large meal.*
- *Work an exercise program to improve endurance; such programs have the bonus of getting you in shape for sex—all the more reason to start that walking program (see pages 62–65).*

Of course, sexual activity doesn't have to mean just sexual intercourse. There are many ways for two consenting adults to please each other sexually, and now might be the time to explore some alternatives.

Conserving your energy also means changing your way of thinking. Don't permit yourself to be overburdened by either possessions or old habits. You will be amazed when you learn how many energy-wasters you can eliminate with no noticeable loss—and considerable relief. Just one example is packing for vacations. Do you really need to take all those clothes?

Each COPD patient is unique. No two have exactly the same needs. Following are some suggestions that may help you greatly and others that may seem nonsensical to you. Each has helped at least one person with COPD.

Waking Up

This is a difficult time for many people with COPD, and if you are not feeling particularly well, it can be a real chore. Here are some hints:

- Soft music is much more pleasant than an alarm.
- Try some stretching and relaxing exercises while still lying down. These help to get your body in gear for the day.
- Making a bed is a demanding household task; if you must do it yourself, try this: half-make your

bed while you are still in it. Pull the top sheet and blanket up on one side and smooth them out. Exit from the unmade side, which is then easy to finish.

- If you find that a bedspread is a luxury that only adds work, go without it.

- An aid to making your bed while still in it is to mark the center of each sheet and blanket in a small permanent way, such as with a colored stitch or pen mark, on the top hem. While you are still sitting on your bed it is easy to line up the marks in the center. When you do get up, everything will be in the right place.

- Before getting all the way up, do some of your dressing while sitting on the edge of your bed. Every night leave your robe and slippers or shoes, socks, and underwear where they are easy to reach. This will require less effort in the morning.

- If you share quarters with another person, persuade him or her to let you have the bureau drawers that are easiest to reach. This will save you from having to bend.

- If you have a room to yourself, put the most often used items, such as socks and underwear, in the most convenient places and store the seldom

used items in the faraway bottom drawers and
top closet shelves.

Bathing

Bathing need not be an ordeal. Following are some
energy-saving hints:

- If for some reason you find a shower or tub bath
  too demanding, get a bath stool that is water-
  proof and goes right into the tub.[2] For bathing,
  use a hand spray. You may find bathing this way
  very pleasant.
- It is not necessary to get instantly wet all over to
  get clean. A "basin bath" can be taken in place of
  a tub bath and is a lot less taxing.
- A nice, long terry robe will eliminate the effort
  of drying altogether. Just blot.
- When excess humidity bothers you, leave the
  bathroom door open and be sure to use your bathroom exhaust fan if you have one. If you feel
  weak, don't take a bath or shower when you are
  alone.
- If you use oxygen, pass the tube over the shower
  curtain rod to keep it out of the way.

2. Many time- and energy-saving products and devices are available for people
with COPD. One of the most comprehensive sources for such items is Sears, which
offers a free catalog. Use it to learn what's available. It is available by calling (800)
326-1750. Otherwise, products can be ordered through your local pharmacy.

- Shaving or applying makeup is much easier if you have a low mirror so you can sit down while doing it.
- It is probably okay to remove the nasal cannula briefly to wash your face, shave, or apply makeup. Check with your doctor.

Grooming Hints

When examining your grooming habits, look not only at the processes but also at the products.

- When you have lung disease, strong scents can be irritating and unpleasant. Try to avoid toiletries that are too heavily perfumed. They may leave you gasping.
- Avoid elaborate hairstyles that will need tiresome setting and extended use of handheld dryers.
- Also, and most important, using aerosols and sprays, except as medicines prescribed by a physician, may add to your respiratory problems. There are many liquid or gel hair dressings and roll-on or solid deodorants to choose from, and many of these products are available unscented.
- If you are troubled by occasional accidental loss of urine brought on by coughing, overexertion, or stress, small, flat sanitary pads with adhesive backs may help keep you dry.

Dressing

You may feel that it is a good idea to finish dressing before breakfast. It gets the day off to a good start.

- Avoid wearing anything that restricts chest or abdominal expansion, including tight belts, bras, panty hose, and girdles. If a choice must be made between style and comfort, opt for comfort every time.
- Suspenders are generally more comfortable than a belt.
- Place your underwear inside your pants and put both on together.
- Slip-on shoes eliminate bending over to tie shoelaces. Your favorite lace-up shoes can even be converted to slip-ons by using elastic shoelaces. Putting on any kind of shoe is much easier if you use a long (twelve to eighteen inches) shoehorn.
- Avoid tight neck bands. Although some gentlemen still prefer neckties, an open neck with a loosely tied scarf, kerchief, or bolo tie is attractive and much more comfortable than a necktie. Another option is a colored T-shirt under an open-neck sport shirt.
- Cotton underclothing is more comfortable

than synthetic. Some nationwide mail-order houses carry complete lines of specialty cotton undergarments.

- "Long johns" are back in style for both sexes. Some of the new colored varieties, originally made for skiers, are quite attractive. They are most comfortable when worn under wide-legged slacks.
- If you are not too active and sit a lot, a large shawl is terrific for occasional shivers and is much easier to put on and take off than a sweater.

Medications

If you take pills, you'll need to get organized about dosages and refills.

- Try using a pillbox with a separate compartment for each day of the week.
- If you are taking many pills, lay out a day's supply each morning.
- Save the one-ounce plastic cups with snap-on lids that fast-food places use for condiments such as ketchup. (Get friends to save some for you.) Have one cup for each pill-taking occasion during the day. Label or mark each cup with the time the contents are to be taken.

- Keep pills in plain sight with a clock nearby and a pad and pencil handy to keep track of your pill taking.
- Remember to store pills away from heat and moisture.
- Whenever you get a new medicine or a refill from the pharmacy, figure out how long the supply will last and mark on a calendar the time to reorder. This may save you from running out of medication in the middle of the night or on a holiday weekend.
- NEVER USE ANYONE ELSE'S MEDICINE! Medicines affect each of us differently. Two people may have the same disease and the same symptoms and yet respond to the same medicine in entirely different ways.
- Never hesitate to ask for more information regarding your medicine or to tell your doctor when your medicine does not seem to be working for you. Never change the dosage without your doctor's permission.
- If you are experiencing unwanted side effects from any medication, contact your doctor or pharmacist immediately.

Respiratory Therapy

If it is necessary for you to take breathing treatments at home, try to keep all of your equipment in a convenient place where it can be left between treatments. Being near a bathroom or kitchen where it will be easy to clean equipment is helpful; but of course, if you take treatments during the night, the first consideration may be to have your equipment near your bed.

- An ideal arrangement is to have a small table with a drawer or a flat-topped desk in front of a window. Outside the window might be a good place to put a bird feeder. It is nice to have something to watch, read, or listen to while taking a treatment. One word of caution—when you are finished, don't leave any medication sitting in the sun.
- You may find it difficult to listen to anything with a machine going. A radio or TV set with a small earphone attachment will solve this problem.
- Have a clock handy to time your treatments.
- If you must measure a medication with an eyedropper, wait for the air bubbles to go away before starting to measure.
- An excellent place to store small pieces of equipment such as tubes, medicine cups, and mouthpieces is in one or two food storage boxes with

lock tops. A good size is about 6" x 8" x 2½". These will fit in a small drawer out of sight, and parts can be sterilized and soaked right in the container.

- Keep all equipment clean and sterilized as directed. Don't worry if a friend has been taught different methods. Several different processes yield the same end result.

- When you disassemble your equipment to clean it after a treatment, you may find that the plastic hose is difficult to pull loose. Try pulling it off while the machine is still running. The added "push" of the compressor will help loosen the hose.

- If you are using a mechanical nebulizer and feel you are not getting enough mist, hand-tighten the hose coupling. Occasionally vibrations cause it to work loose.

- Any small piece of equipment with a motor or compressor will be much quieter if you put some kind of a thick pad under it. Folded fabric or newspaper may suffice.

- If your equipment has an air filter, remember to change it occasionally.

- Most medical equipment used at home can be purchased. In many cases this may be cheaper than monthly rental, but you will be responsible for repairs. Ask your supplier and compare.

Oxygen

Make an appointment to have your supplier come visit you to explain all the technical aspects of the operation of your equipment. Get an emergency phone number and a list of procedures to follow in case of malfunctions or concerns about the equipment. However, since oxygen itself is a prescribed drug, questions about amount and usage should be answered by your physician.

• Some portable oxygen units (oxygen walkers) come equipped with a loose scale on the side for measuring the weight of the liquid oxygen. Those who use this type of system over a period of time often learn to estimate the weight fairly accurately. In this case the scale can be removed, leaving a leather loop with snap in place. The oxygen tubing can be threaded through this loop to eliminate some of the strain on the point of attachment of the tube to the pack. This helps prevent the tubing from being accidentally disconnected. The same method can be used to temporarily shorten the tube by looping it through several times.

- It is important to find out approximately how long each portable unit supply will last you. Learn to time your outings so that you don't run short of oxygen.
- If you have been out with a portable liquid unit and return home with no immediate plans to go out again soon, you can transfer your long house tubing to the portable unit to use up the remaining oxygen it holds. This utilizes oxygen that would otherwise only leak away.
- Change nasal cannulas fairly often, particularly if the prongs become soiled or uncomfortable. Many suppliers replace them at no cost.
- Don't be embarrassed by the occasional attention your oxygen unit and tubing may attract. Most people know what it is and give it no more thought than they would a hearing aid. Others, who may not be familiar with this equipment, are interested in learning what it is. They appreciate your taking the time to explain what it does and why you must use it.

Work at Home or Abroad

This is where some of us temporarily bog down. Each person with COPD must find his or her own work ethic. Try not to rush. Many good books and paintings have been literally years in the making. If you don't feel like building a World Trade Center today, how about trying to lay a couple of bricks? There are many different jobs we can do. Don't be afraid to start small. It beats not starting at all.

Lifting and Toting

Housework can't be avoided, but it can be made easier. Following are some tips:

- Get yourself a small utility cart, the kind with three shelves. As you move about doing chores, use your cart to carry everything that needs to be transferred from one place to another. Pick up last night's newspaper, some soiled clothes for the laundry, a couple of used dishes, books to go back to the library, clean towels for the bathroom, and so forth.
- Try to travel in a circle, and avoid going back and forth. Using a cart and working in a circle are very effective whether you live in a single room or a two-story house (have a cart on each floor).
- If you do live in a single room or a small apartment, it is especially important to maintain reasonable order. Living in untidy quarters can be depressing. Try to stay on top of your chores and create a pleasant ambiance for yourself. It will make you feel better.

• Carrying things downstairs is not a problem for most of us. Carrying them up may be a different story. If you must carry things upstairs, try this: On an exhale, lift your burden two or three steps and put it down to rest. Climb two or three steps, and rest again. Repeat. This may be a little slow, but it is possible to do the job without knocking yourself out.

For those with advanced COPD, a one-floor living plan may work best. If you have less severe COPD, stairs are good exercise, though it is a good idea to have a chair to sit on or a table to lean on when you reach the top.

Cleaning Tools

The tools you use for cleaning can make all the difference in the world. Many people with COPD find the following tools and hints helpful:

• One of the handiest gadgets is a pair of pick-up tongs (they look like giant scissors) used for retrieving objects from hard-to-reach places. Most medical supply houses stock these. One type of pick-up tongs expands in a crisscross fashion. They are made of metal or wood and make it possible to pick up very small objects without bending. They are marvelous but hard to find. If you are lucky enough to find them, try slipping a small piece of rubber tubing over each end; this makes it easier to grasp things.

- Another pick-up device is a magnet on a short string. This will stick to your cart, so you will always have it with you. It's great for retrieving thumbtacks, lost hairpins, and the like.

- A small hand vacuum is more convenient for spot cleanups than a full-size one, and it can be placed on your cart. If you must use a full-size vacuum, use a newer machine with a disposable bag, and remove it with extreme care.

- Sweeping and feather-dusting are out, but if you do feel compelled to use a broom or dry mop, protect yourself by wrapping the working end in a damp cloth.

- Even with precautions, housework is apt to stir up dust. If you find you must do a dusty job, the best idea is to use a mask (available from good hardware stores).

- Around the house the "no aerosol" rule applies— no ifs, ands, or buts. Also avoid strong odors and fumes given off by kitchen and bathroom cleaners, any of which may contain lye, ammonia, or other chemicals.

- Avoid using anything harmful that can vaporize, such as kerosene, mothballs, and solvents. Also avoid powders as much as possible; if they must be used, handle with extreme care.

- Pets, which can provide much-needed companionship, are not a good idea if your COPD has an asthma component, because of shedding and dander (the dandruff-like substance from the coat or feathers of animals).
- Have good ventilation and an adequate supply of fresh air at all times.

A Friend in Need

If you can't afford a housekeeper—and not many people can—don't hesitate to ask for help from friends or family. You'd be surprised to find out just how many people are willing to pitch in. Often, people with COPD stubbornly resist the urge to ask for assistance. Remember, if you're doing the right kind of "work" to improve your relationship with yourself, others, and your Higher Power (see chapter 2), chances are the people around you will be eager to lend a hand. They may be waiting to be asked.

In the Kitchen

The kitchen means not just cleaning, but cooking. Following are some tips for both:

- Don't try to get everything done at once; instead, set small goals. Almost all jobs can be divided into sections. For instance, clean the top shelf of the refrigerator today and the bottom shelf tomorrow or next week.
- Plan your meals when you are neither hungry nor tired. Light, well-balanced meals are too important to leave to impulse.
- A number of small meals is better than a few large ones. The more room the stomach takes up, the less room there is for air in the lungs. Also, the larger the meal, the more prolonged the digestion, which draws blood and oxygen to the stomach and away from other parts of the body that may need them more.
- Utilize convenience foods when necessary, but remember that many packaged foods have a high salt and sugar content, which may be off-limits if you are on a special diet. Get in the habit of reading labels.
- Keep plenty of water and fruit juices in the refrigerator.
- If you enjoy cooking, it is often almost as easy to make a double or triple amount of your specialties. Freeze the excess in meal-size containers and enjoy some cooking-free days.
- When cooking, always use your exhaust fan or

make sure there is good ventilation. Exhaust fans should be ventilated outside.

- If you are bothered by the heat, try using a small portable fan when cooking or ironing. These are available from most appliance stores. In fact, a portable fan is useful in any room, not only to cool you off but also to help overcome the shortness of breath brought on by exertion or stress. It is also useful for blowing offensive or irritating odors away from you, should the need arise. In fact, a portable fan may deserve a place on your cart.
- When tidying up after a meal, assemble all items that need putting away in the refrigerator in one spot. Then sit down in front of the refrigerator and put them away.
- After scrubbing pots and pans, store the ones you use most often on the stove for easy access. Instead of putting your dishes and utensils away, reset the table for your next meal.

Gardening

If you enjoy gardening, there are a number of ways to make it easier.

- First, get a riding mower, preferably with a self-starter.

- An old-fashioned but effective tool is a small floral or scuffle hoe. These are light and easy to handle. Cut down weeds while they are still small and leave them where they fall; they make good mulch.
- Some other easy-to-handle, lightweight tools are a seven-inch-wide floral rake; a three-pronged cultivator with a handle about three feet long, and a nylon garden hose that rolls up flat on its own reel. One of these hoses, fifty feet long with its reel, weighs only two and a half pounds and can be carried in one hand.
- If bending over cuts off your wind, try sitting down on a folding stool. Use a long-handled spear-type weeder, a clam rake about eighteen inches long for leaves, and your pick-up scissors or tongs, which are useful for removing garden debris from the ground. Both the tools and the folding stool can be carried in a shallow garden basket.
- Here's how to make an easy flower garden. In the fall, gather as many seeds as possible from easy-to-grow, hardy annuals. Store them in airtight bags. In the spring, sow each kind separately, scattering by hand in prepared beds. Rake in and tamp lightly. When the plants come up, hoe down all but a few. What remains will give

you a nice display without the hard work of
transplanting seedlings.
- If you live where there is no space for your own
garden, you may be able to get a window box or
several shelves for plants inside the window.
Even in a limited space, gardening can be a
tremendously rewarding pursuit.

Going Out

This is a good place to repeat that all COPD people are
different in many ways. One way is in your reaction to
weather. Some like it hot, some like it cold, some
damp, some dry. The point is that if it is your kind of
day, try to get out and enjoy it.

- One thing that does bother all people with COPD
considerably is air pollution. Find out where you
can get a daily air quality report for your area,
and consult it when making your plans for the
day.
- Before leaving for an outing, lay out your comfortable clothes and slippers, prepare some juice
in a handy thermos, set out whatever utensils
you will need for your evening meal, or turn
down your bed for a quick nap—whatever makes
you feel good. Then homecoming will be more
than just a relief; it will be a pleasure.

- Try to get yourself a warm, lightweight coat for winter. Down is ideal. A heavy winter coat can wear you out before you are out the front door.
- In cold weather, also don a long, warm scarf. If conditions get too cold or windy, wear the scarf across your nose. Some COPD sufferers, however, prefer a cold-weather mask. You can now get one made of soft sponge that is quite comfortable to wear. Those of you who walk a lot may find that a cane-seat, or shooting stick, is a real help. It provides an all-in-one cane to lean on and a small seat if you feel like resting.

Riding and Driving

If you have trouble getting from point A to point B, it matters not whether the problem arises in your legs or your lungs. If you have trouble walking, you are entitled to a handicapped parking permit. It is simple to obtain in most places. Write to your State Motor Vehicle Department for an application. When you use a handicapped parking space, make sure you display your permit; this is required by law in many states.

- If someone is helping you with errands, you probably have to sit in the car for fairly long periods of time. Make up a kit for yourself and keep it in the car. In a shopping bag, for instance, include a pad and pencil, a paperback book or two, tissues, a package of premoistened wipes, and whatever else suits your needs. It also helps to carry a large piece of cardboard to use as a sunscreen if necessary.

- A coffee can with a snap-on plastic lid will work as an emergency urinal.
- If you do drive alone and find that you must put gas in your car yourself, try to get upwind from the pump so you do not breathe in the fumes.
- For drivers with breathing problems, a cellular phone may be a necessity. Try to imagine changing a tire, walking to the next off-ramp to call for help, or hiking a long distance carrying a can of gas.
- When driving, practice doing breathing exercises while waiting for red lights to change—it beats fuming. Take a couple of minutes or even seconds to do breathing exercises whenever you come to a natural stopping place: a red light, a stop sign, or a crosswalk.

Traveling

If you plan an intercity trip, think of taking a bus, which will usually take you to the middle of town where other local transportation is available. On interstate buses, the federal smoking laws are generally observed. Sit in the front, and if you have any special problems, tell the driver. Following are some traveling tips:

- When you must travel alone, travel light. Get a small suitcase on wheels. There are also wheel-equipped suitcase carriers, which are effective but clumsy (and just something else to carry around).
- Subways are generally an undesirable environment for anyone with respiratory problems. Most subways and elevated train lines can be accessed only by long and exhausting stair climbs. This may be made many times more difficult by being caught in rush-hour crowds which force you to move much faster than is comfortable. In addition, the air in many older subway systems can be choked with dust. Use whatever surface transportation is available.
- Whenever possible, avoid any kind of travel during rush hours so you can move at your own speed if you are driving and find a seat if you are using public transportation.

Shopping

Whether you consider shopping a chore or a pleasure, it can still be tiring. Following are some tips to make your shopping trip easier:

- If you are going shopping with an oxygen carrier, find a shopping cart on your way into the store. Keep your oxygen unit in the cart while you shop.
- When you go shopping, pick an off day and hour (not Saturday at high noon). You will be able to move at a leisurely pace and can avoid being jostled.
- Avoid crowds in general, particularly indoors. Aside from the fact that the air may be smoky and generally unpleasant, you run a high risk of having someone sneeze or cough nearby.
- Don't be afraid to ask someone to stop smoking near you. We all have a right to breathe smoke-free air, as most people are beginning to realize.
- In many areas there are no-smoking laws. Familiarize yourself with these; and if you are in a store or restaurant where these laws are not being observed, speak to the manager. Don't forget, you are the customer.
- Shopping for clothing, especially dresses and slacks, can be exhausting even if you're in the best of health. Know your measurements (write them down) and carry a small rolled-up tape measure with you. If you see something you like, check with the tape to see if it will fit before you buy. Make sure that if it isn't satisfactory, it can be returned.

- When you have a fairly large grocery order, have all the perishables, such as milk and frozen foods, packed in a separate bag. When you get home, you can put away whatever needs refrigeration. Leave the rest for later when you feel more energetic or when someone can lend a hand.
- It won't hurt to wash your hands extra well when you get home. It is now known that colds are spread by hands as well as through the air.

Rest and Recreation

One of the most important and lasting pleasures any of us can have is the company of good friends. The mobile society we live in often makes it difficult to keep in touch with old acquaintances. Many of us live far from our birthplaces and early ties, and we sometimes feel that after a certain age it is hard to start making new friends. On the contrary, you have many opportunities to strike up friendships. Consider the following possibilities:

- You may already have developed relationships with others in a Twelve Step group, such as Nicotine Anonymous. Another way to make friends with whom you can share common interests and problems is to join a Respiratory Club.

If you can't find such a group, get in touch with your local Lung Association or your hospital respiratory department.

How to Get Help Quickly When It May Be Needed

- *The buddy phone system can be a big help and provide a special feeling of security.*
- *Make arrangements to have a friend or relative call at the same time every day to make sure you are okay. If you plan to be out, let him or her know ahead of time to save needless concern.*
- *Get to know neighbors who can see your windows and arrange a signal they can see. For instance, if a shade is pulled down every evening or a certain lamp is lit, it is a sign that you are okay. If they don't see the signal, ask your neighbors to investigate.*
- *If you live in an apartment, let the neighbors on all sides of you know that if they hear you pounding, you need help.*

- Somewhere near you is someone who needs your friendship and help too. Once you have gotten in touch with others, you will be amazed to find how rewarding it can be.

- You may have forgotten about board games. You probably have some around your house that haven't been used in a long time—checkers, Parcheesi, Monopoly, Scrabble, etc. And don't forget card games like whist, pinochle, rummy, or canasta.
- If you are a chess buff, you might enjoy joining a chess club. It is also fun to play games through the mail, e-mail, or over the phone.
- When you need time to yourself, try solitaire—it can be very relaxing. Several books on the market describe numerous versions of solitaire. Try learning a new game or two.
- Jigsaw puzzles can keep you focused and provide a real sense of accomplishment.
- Do you like to read? Build up a supply of paperbacks for days when you can't get out to the library. Many libraries have a give-away box of paperbacks. If yours doesn't, ask the librarian to start one. You can also get good books cheaply at flea markets or garage sales, and you can trade books with friends, neighbors, and relatives. If you can't get out, ask if your library has a home delivery service.
- Is there a skill you have always wanted to learn or a class you've always wanted to take? Now is the

time. Many local schools have adult classes in the evening on a staggering assortment of subjects. If you prefer to learn in the relaxing atmosphere of your home, there are literally hundreds of correspondence courses to choose from, from beekeeping to weather forecasting. Distance learning courses are also available on the Internet.

- If you have always wanted to learn a language, try a home-study course with tapes. This is more fun if you find someone to practice your new language with. An e-mail correspondent or telephone or pen pal might be just the thing.

- If you find your previous hobbies too demanding, try a moderated version for the time being. Cabinetmakers may find great pleasure in making scale-model furniture; machinists might enjoy making a scale-model locomotive or assembling a clock; dressmakers could make and dress period-costume dolls.

- Is a rambunctious dog too much to handle? Try a small, quiet cat. If allergies forbid either, tropical fish, while not very affectionate, are beautiful and fascinating. They are also very low maintenance, provided you can get someone to clean the tank periodically. A bird feeder near your favorite window can provide hours of pleasure. If, for some reason, none of these are possible, a large stuffed animal has its uses as a confidant, punching bag, or pillow.

- Needlework of various kinds can provide both relaxation and pleasure. At least half of the world's champion knitters and crocheters have been men. Try it—you might like it.
- If you like to paint, try watercolors for a change of pace. They are lightweight, odorless, and fast-drying. To develop a technique for using them, try some of the new coloring books for adults. These are really great fun for everyone, not just artists.
- This may be a good time to learn to play a musical instrument like piano or guitar. (The wind instruments are out, however—no tubas!)
- Nowadays almost anything you could possibly want to buy can be purchased through the mail and the Internet. So let your fingers do the walking not only through the phone book but also through a whole world of mail-order catalogs. Many pleasant evenings can be spent sitting in your favorite (not too soft) easy chair and shopping or "surfing the Net" in search of good buys.

Bed

After all these activities, you'll be ready for bed. Following are some tips to make your nights as comfortable as your days.

- Go to bed in easy stages so that you arrive there relaxed, not worn out. For example, put on your nightclothes and a comfortable robe, and then read or watch TV for a while.
- Plan your sleeping area so that everything you may need will be handy, the most important items being a light and telephone. Have any emergency numbers you think you might need taped to the phone (make sure they're easy to read).
- Other helpful items include a clock radio with an earplug for late-night listening (if you have a sleeping companion), medication, a glass of water and a small snack, and a urinal in a safe, easy-to-reach place. (One little-known fact is that there are also urinals made for women.)
- An electric blanket is a must. No other blanket is necessary. They are lightweight, comfortable, and make bed-making a cinch. Remember to follow all safety precautions.
- A night-light lessens the possibility of being disoriented if you awaken suddenly and helps you locate things you may need in a hurry.

• A light that throws the time on the ceiling and numerous small lamps that plug directly into a wall outlet are now available. Watching a lava lamp may also relax you and make you go to sleep. Best of all is a lighted aquarium which, in a darkened room, is enchanting. Some find this is a perfect time to do some muscle-relaxing exercises.

So pull your nightcap (no kidding) down over your ears, say your prayers (if you are so inclined), and go to sleep. Pleasant dreams.

CHAPTER FIVE

Surgical Options for Advanced COPD

If you have advanced COPD, you might decide after much thought and prayer to have surgery for your condition. The decision is not an easy one. The risks are high and the outcome uncertain. You weigh the options given to you by your doctor. In communion with your Higher Power, you decide whether it feels right to take this major step.

Surgical options for COPD are limited because of the destruction of the architecture of the lung. Two main surgical options exist for people with COPD: lung transplantation and lung-reduction surgery. Because of the risks involved, both procedures are performed only in people with severe, or end-stage, COPD.

Lung Transplantation

Of the two procedures, lung transplantation is more tried and tested—single and double transplants have been performed for the last fifteen to twenty years. However, lung transplantation is often not a suitable option for those with advanced COPD. These people are typically elderly and have other serious medical conditions associated with their lung disease, including heart problems. For these men and women, the operation itself and the postoperative regimen to prevent rejection may be life-threatening. On the other hand, for some COPD sufferers, a transplant is their only hope of reaching old age.

The Procedure

The goal of a lung transplantation is to replace diseased lungs with healthy lungs obtained from a compatible donor who has just died. One or both lungs may be replaced.

After general anesthesia is administered, an incision is made in the recipient's chest, and the chest is spread open. A heart-lung machine keeps the patient alive. The surgeon then cuts the lungs free of the connecting bronchial tubes and blood vessels and removes them. The donor lungs are positioned and sewn into place. Blood vessels and bronchial tubes are surgically connected. The chest muscles are closed and the skin stitched, or sutured, shut.

Stitches are usually removed one week after surgery. The average hospital stay after this procedure is three weeks. When the operation is successful, recovery time is six months.

The procedure is approximately equal in pain and trauma to open-heart surgery. However, it is not done nearly as often as open-heart surgery because of the relative lack of donor lungs and the need for a very close match. The average cost for lung transplantation is $300,000.

Drawbacks

Unfortunately, the statistics are grim for people who undergo lung transplants. Approximately 10 percent of recipients die on the operating table or in immediate recovery from trauma or infection. During the first year after surgery, about 30 percent of patients die because their bodies reject the transplanted lungs or they succumb to other diseases because their natural immunity is lowered by powerful antirejection medications. In patients who live beyond the first year, the average duration of survival is five years.

Benefits

Patients whose lung transplants are successful can expect to breathe almost normally after they have recovered from the surgery. No longer will they need supplemental oxygen to get through the day. Nor will they suffer the many symptoms associated with advanced

COPD—sleeplessness, headaches, irritability, and lack of concentration. Most people are able to resume a moderate exercise program.

Lung-Reduction Surgery

Emphysema-dominant COPD causes the lungs to overinflate. Eventually, the lungs fill the chest cavity, which then has difficulty expanding.

Lung-reduction surgery is a fairly recent therapeutic option for emphysema-dominant COPD sufferers and one that is potentially more suitable for greater numbers of people than lung transplantation. By removing the most diseased portions of the lungs (about 15 to 30 percent of the total volume of the lungs), the operation gives the chest cavity and lungs room to expand when a breath is taken.

Also known as *reduction pneumoplasty, lung shaving,* and *lung contouring,* the procedure is performed on patients with end-stage emphysema-dominant COPD.

The Procedure

A series of inch-long incisions is made between the patient's ribs. A tiny "live-action" video camera is inserted through one of these incisions so the surgeons can watch what they are doing. Through the incisions, a surgeon inserts a cutting tool or laser to trim diseased tissue from the lung. Tissue that is still functioning is left intact. Usually about 15 to 30 percent of the lung is cut away.

Whenever possible, this kind of surgery is performed on both lungs to provide maximum improvement in lung function.

The minimally invasive technique used to perform lung-reduction surgery (known as *thorascopy*) provides the surgeons with a better view of the patient's lungs than when the chest is opened in conventional lung surgery.

Drawbacks

The risks of lung-reduction surgery are about half that of transplantation, but the improvements are not as pronounced. The cost is between $35,000 and $60,000, depending on the particular doctor and hospital.

Although lung-reduction surgery looks promising, the medical profession is being appropriately cautious about the procedure. And because it is still considered experimental, insurance does not cover the cost. However, lung-reduction surgery is expected to eventually become an accepted and common way to treat end-stage emphysema-dominant COPD.

Benefits

At present, most patients experience greater than a 20 percent increase in lung function (measured by maximal breath tests), and a significant number of patients improve lung function by more than 50 percent. Patients who undergo successful lung-reduction surgery can expect to experience significant improvement in their condition—better breathing, concentration, and sleep patterns, as well as fewer headaches and sexual dysfunctions.

National Study to Ascertain Reduction Surgery Effectiveness

A major clinical trial sponsored by Medicare and the National Institutes of Health is under way to confirm the safety and effectiveness of lung-reduction surgery. Known as the National Emphysema Treatment Trial (NETT), the study will also try to determine how best to select patients for the procedure and how to assess the different surgical techniques being used. The seven-year study, which began in October 1997, is being conducted at eighteen centers specializing in lung surgery. All participants have been selected for the study.

As medical science becomes more sophisticated, surgical techniques for COPD may improve. Future technological advances may improve the success rates for surgical procedures, but for now, surgery remains a last resort. COPD treatments such as exercise and taking proper medication remain the cornerstone of effective management of COPD.

Remember that if you are following the principles of the Twelve Steps, you "turned over" control of your disease to your Higher Power and undertook the responsibility to cooperate in doing everything you can to help manage your disease. In part this means being as healthy as possible in anticipation of the day when you may need surgery.

CHAPTER SIX

Complementary and Alternative Treatments for COPD

You have turned over control of your disease to a Higher Power. Your role now is to cooperate with that Power by doing whatever you can to care for yourself. That includes finding out what treatments are available that may help alleviate or improve your condition, even those outside the realm of "conventional" medicine.

Complementary and alternative medicines are treatments and health care approaches not taught widely in Western medical schools, not generally used in hospitals, and not usually reimbursed by medical insurance. The term covers a wide range of ancient healing philosophies, approaches, and therapies.

The terms *complementary* and *alternative* are not interchangeable. Therapies used *in conjunction with* conventional medicine are referred to as complementary. Therapies used *instead of* conventional medicine are considered to be alternative.

Certain complementary and alternative approaches are based on familiar principles of Western medicine, but many have quite different origins. Many therapies remain far outside the realm of accepted Western medicine, while others have been embraced by large segments of society.

Consider, for instance, the ancient Chinese medical practice of acupuncture. Once considered quite bizarre in the West, the procedure is now increasingly used by ordinary Americans to treat medical conditions, to relieve stress, and even to ease symptoms during nicotine withdrawal. The same may be said for herbal medicine, as evidenced by the television commercials for and widespread availability of products containing echinacea, ginseng, and Saint-John's-wort.

It is a measure of society's interest in alternatives to conventional medicine that led the government-run National Institutes of Health (NIH) to create the Office of Alternative Medicine (OAM) in 1992. OAM facilitates research and evaluation of unconventional medical practices and disseminates this information to the public. Its budget in 1998 was $20 million. You can obtain a classification of forty-seven complementary and alternative medical health care practices from the OAM. The list is intended to show the diversity of the field and is neither complete nor authoritative.

Many practitioners of conventional health care dispute the claims of alternative and complementary medicine because, by and large, such therapies are not investigated using the same scientific research methods used in conventional medicine. The herbal remedies have neither Food and Drug Administration (FDA) approval nor regulation. The benefits of such treatments, Western-trained doctors argue, are strictly anecdotal; that is, they are based on patient testimonials, not documented results. It is unlikely that alternative and complementary medicine will be fully accepted until its practitioners can produce results based on rigorous research methods dependent upon systematic, explicit, and comprehensive knowledge and skills.

How to Find Out More about Complementary and Alternative Treatments for COPD

Health care providers are becoming more familiar with alternative and complementary treatments, and your doctor may be willing to refer you to such a practitioner. Medical professionals on the whole, however, are suspicious of medical treatments they consider untested, unproven, and thus potentially harmful.

Don't be discouraged if your doctor cannot or will not provide you with the information you want. Good sources of information about particular complementary and alternative medical practices are available in medical libraries, public libraries, and bookstores.

Other resources for complementary and alternative therapies are the twenty-four institutes, centers, and divisions of the NIH. For information from the NIH on COPD itself, call (301) 496-4000 and ask the operator to direct you to the appropriate office.

The advent of the Internet has made research into alternative and complementary medicine much easier—especially for people with chronic illnesses such as COPD whose mobility is restricted. If you have a telephone line and can afford a computer, then the vast resources of the Internet are available to you. If you can't afford a computer, you should be aware that many libraries have computers that are hooked up to the Internet for use by library members. Once you are on-line, access to most medical research resources on the Internet is free. Some sites—such as thriveonline.com—take the latest medical research and "translate" it into information the ordinary person can understand. An excellent on-line source of complementary and alternative medicine is the alternative medicine section of www.healthanswers.com. Lessons in the basics of using the Internet are widely available, and classes may be held at your local library, senior center, or adult learning center.

To find out more about complementary and alternative treatments for COPD, you may also want to ask practitioners of complementary and alternative medicine about their practices. Many practitioners belong to a growing number of professional associations, educational organizations, and research institutions that provide information about complementary and alternative medical practices. A growing number of these organizations have sites on the Internet.

Remember, some of these organizations advocate a specific therapy or treatment but are unable to provide complete and objective health information. Before trying out any treatment, make sure to get as much information as you can and discuss your findings and thoughts with your doctor.

How to Find a Practitioner in Your Area

To find a qualified complementary and/or alternative medical health care practitioner, contact medical regulatory and licensing agencies in your state (your health care provider should be able to provide you with their names). Such regulatory and licensing bodies can provide information about a specific practitioner's credentials and background. Many states license practitioners who provide alternative therapies such as acupuncture, chiropractic services, naturopathy, herbal medicine, homeopathy, and massage therapy.

You also may locate individual practitioners by

asking your health care provider or by contacting a professional association or organization. These organizations can provide names of local practitioners and information about how to determine the quality of a specific practitioner's services.

What to Consider When Choosing a Therapy or Practitioner

The health decisions you make are important, and choosing to explore complementary and alternative treatments is no exception. There are some serious issues you need to address when selecting an alternative or complementary therapy or practitioner. In particular, ask yourself questions about safety and effectiveness of the treatment, the qualifications of the practitioner, and the cost of the therapy.

Is It Safe? Is It Effective?

The therapy should provide relief from the condition for which it is sought—in this case, COPD—and it should not have the ability to cause you harm when used as intended. Unfortunately, less is known about the safety and effectiveness of complementary and alternative products and practices than conventional medicine. So what can you do?

Ask the alternative/complementary health practitioner for evidence of the safety and effectiveness of the practice, treatment, or technology he or she advocates. Request information on new research that either supports or debunks the effectiveness of the treatment, and also ask about any new information about its safety.

You should also ask questions about possible side effects, interactions with other medications you are taking, expected results, and how long the treatment should last.

Make sure the practitioner is aware of all other therapies—both conventional and alternative/complementary—you are using, as this information will probably be necessary to ensure the safety and effectiveness of the treatment plan.

Published information on the safety and effectiveness of particular therapies can be found in scientific journals available at certain public libraries, university libraries, medical libraries, on-line computer services, and the U.S. National Library of Medicine (NLM) at the National Institutes of Health (NIH). As the articles in these journals can be difficult for the layperson to understand, you might find the summary at the beginning of the manuscript, known as the "abstract," the easiest way to gain information from these materials. You can find these scientific articles in the *Index Medicus,* a published resource available in medical and university libraries and some public libraries.

The World Wide Web can be an excellent source of information about the safety and effectiveness of complementary and alternative medicine, although it is important that you learn to differentiate between credible and non-credible sources. This ability to discern comes with time spent using the Internet.

Also try to gain access to people with COPD who have received the treatment you are researching. Remember, though, that anecdotal evidence from other patients is not an accurate measure of the safety and effectiveness of a treatment. Therefore, it should not be the sole criteria for selecting an alternative or complementary therapy. Studies done under controlled conditions by trained medical scientists are the best way to assess a treatment's effectiveness.

What Are the Practitioner's Qualifications?

Research the background, qualifications, and reputation of the practitioner. You can do this by contacting the state or local regulatory body that has jurisdiction over the practice of the therapy you are seeking. Although complementary and alternative medicine is not as strictly regulated as conventional medicine, licensing and accreditation are continually being introduced.

Local and state medical boards may be able to provide information about an individual practitioner's credentials, and consumer affairs departments such as the Better Business Bureau can tell you whether there have been any complaints lodged against that person.

How Much Does It Cost?

Your health insurer or the practitioner should be able to tell you whether a particular therapy is covered by insurance. However, most complementary and alternative treatments are not covered by health insurance. Patients usually have to pay the entire amount of the therapy. Thus cost is a very important factor for people seeking alternative and complementary medical treatments.

"Shop around" to find out what different practitioners charge for the same service. Although cost shouldn't be the sole criteria for selection, knowing what a variety of practitioners charge will give you some idea of what is appropriate. The same professional and regulatory bodies that can provide information on safety and effectiveness should be able to provide approximate cost guidelines.

Specific Complementary and Alternative Treatments for COPD

It is beyond the scope of this book to describe each and every nonconventional treatment for COPD. The following, however, are some of the most common alternative and complementary therapeutic modalities used to treat respiratory disorders that might involve chronic bronchitis, emphysema, or combinations of both.

Herbal Remedies

Herbal medicines are the forerunners of modern pharmaceuticals. Approximately one-quarter of all drugs prescribed by doctors have active ingredients derived from plant medicines. Even aspirin is herbal in origin—it is a derivative of willow tree bark.

The widespread use of herbal medicines declined with the advent of synthetic versions of traditional medicines, which have proven more potent. However, because of possible side effects and the high costs associated with modern drugs, many people have turned to the herbal "roots" of modern medicine.

It is important to remember that herbs are medicines; and, as with any medicine, it's important to know how to take them, how frequently, in what dosages, and how they will interact with your prescription and nonprescription drugs as well as with other herbs. There are plenty of resources on the market that describe how to use herbal medicine. However, it's a good idea to ask for advice from health professionals. You may want to start with MDs and RNs who have an interest in herbal remedies and their implications for people with COPD. Be sure to ask them about side effects or possible interactions with any drugs you may be taking, including caffeine.

Hydrotherapy

The use of cold or hot water to treat a variety of conditions is known as *hydrotherapy.* Hydrotherapy boosts immunity by stimulating lymphatic fluid and increasing blood circulation. Drinking water also flushes unwelcome substances out of our bodies.

Forms of Hydrotherapy

To help relieve symptoms of COPD, water can be used in steam treatments, in cold or hot compresses, or simply ingested from a glass.

What May Be Effective

Drinking eight glasses of water a day will loosen the secretions in your lungs.

A cold-water pack on your chest may relieve congestion, while a hot-water compress on your back between your shoulder blades may reduce coughing.

Inhaling steam can help loosen phlegm in your lungs. First, fill a sink with boiling water. Keeping your eyes closed, drape a towel over your head and inhale the steam for two to five minutes. To further ease breathing and help relieve nasal congestion, try adding a few drops of one or more essential oils into the water.

Before You Start Hydrotherapy

Although some health care practitioners take a particular interest in hydrotherapy, there is no specialty in this area. You can do it yourself, so long as you use a little common sense. Some day-spas also offer forms of hydrotherapy.

Vitamin and Mineral Therapy

The human diet contains numerous vitamins and minerals, many of which would benefit people with COPD if they took them in greater amounts than are available in their normal diet.

Forms of Vitamin and Mineral Therapy

Vitamin and mineral supplements are usually taken in pill form.

What May Be Effective

Garlic capsules can help prevent infection. Vitamins A and C can help strengthen the immune system and help heal inflamed lungs. The mineral magnesium can strengthen the respiratory muscles and therefore reduce the tendency of the bronchial tubes to go into spasm.

Before You Start Vitamin and Mineral Therapy

Taken in excessive doses, most vitamins and minerals will cause unwelcome, and possibly dangerous, side effects, ranging from insomnia to diarrhea and, in rare instances, death. Consult your doctor, a registered dietitian, and/or a qualified nutritionist before starting to take vitamin and mineral supplements for your COPD. At the very least, educate yourself on the subject of vitamin and mineral therapy through the many written and electronic resources presently available.

Complementary or alternative treatments should not be a substitute for any COPD treatments prescribed by your doctor. Before you use a complementary or alternative treatment, thoroughly discuss this decision with your doctor.

Pulmonary Rehabilitation/ Wellness Facilities

This directory of pulmonary rehabilitation facilities was compiled by Bill Horden from a number of sources and was accurate at the time of publication. Both the author and publisher are grateful to Mr. Horden for his permission to reprint this material.

The directory is comprised of multidisciplinary programs—those more likely to treat the "whole" patient and provide the education essential to better manage the disease.

There are many rehabilitation programs that are not considered multidisciplinary. They should, however, be given careful consideration. Many non-multidisciplinary programs offer a free initial consultation and are excellent sources of information.

CANADA

ONTARIO

Grand River Hospital (Freeport Health Centre)
3570 King Street East
Kitchener, Ontario N2A 2W1
Canada
(519) 749-4300, extension 7309 or 7434

UNITED STATES OF AMERICA

ALABAMA

Mobile Infirmary Medical Center
Pulmonary Rehabilitation Education Program (PREP)
192 Louiselle Street
Mobile, AL 36607
(334) 431-4187

Montclair-Baptist Medical Center
720 Montclair Road
Birmingham, AL 35213
(205) 599-4500

Princeton Baptist Medical Center
701 Princeton Avenue Southwest
Birmingham, AL 35211-1399
(205) 783-7460
http://www.baptistmedical.org

ARKANSAS

Baptist Medical Center
9601 I-630, Exit 7
Little Rock, AR 72205
(501) 202-1805

CALIFORNIA

Barlow Respiratory Hospital
2000 Stadium Way
Los Angeles, CA 90026
(213) 250-4200, extension 3153
http://www.barlow2000.org

A highly specialized facility providing both inpatient
and outpatient acute-care, especially the weaning of
patients from prolonged mechanical ventilation.

Beach City's Ambulatory Care Center
514 North Prospect Avenue
Redondo Beach, CA 90277
(310) 937-1979

Casa Colina Hospital
255 East Bonita Avenue
Pomona, CA 91767
(909) 596-7733

Citrus Valley Medical Center
210 West San Bernardino Road
Covina, CA 91723
(626) 331-7331

Dominican Hospital
"Lifestyle Management Programs"
1555 Soquel Drive
Santa Cruz, CA 95065
(831) 457-7077

Hoag Memorial Hospital Presbyterian
One Hoag Drive
P.O. Box 6100
Newport Beach, CA 92658-6100
(949) 760-5831
http://www.hoag.org

Mission Hospital
Pulmonary Rehabilitation and Education Program
27700 Medical Center Road
Mission Viejo, CA 92691
(949) 365-2106

Saint Jude's Medical Center
Pulmonary Wellness Program
101 East Valencia Mesa Drive
Fullerton, CA 92835
(714) 992-3982

COLORADO

National Jewish Research and Medical Center
for Immunology and Respiratory Medicine
1400 Jackson Street
Denver, CO 80206
(303) 398-1783

DELAWARE

Christiana Care Health Services
Riverside Health Care Center
Medical Arts Complex, Suite 103
700 Lea Boulevard
Wilmington, DE 19802
(302) 765-4580

Pulmonary rehabilitation services also available at Christiana Hospital in Newark, Delaware.

FLORIDA

Cape Coral Hospital
Pulmonary Rehabilitation Department
636 Del Prado Boulevard
Cape Coral, FL 33990
(941) 574-2323

GEORGIA

Dekalb Medical Center
2701 North Decatur Road
Decatur, GA 30033
(404) 501-7155

University Hospital
1350 Walton Way
Augusta, GA 30901
(706) 774-5864

IDAHO

Saint Alphonsus Regional Medical Center
1055 North Curtis Road
Boise, ID 83706
(208) 367-3199

ILLINOIS

Rush North Shore Medical Center
9600 Gross Point Road
Skokie, IL 60076
(847) 933-6230

INDIANA

Clarian Health Partners
Methodist Hospital
I-65 at Twenty-first Street
P.O. Box 1367
Indianapolis, IN 46206-1367
(317) 929-5060

Community Hospital East of Indianapolis
1500 North Ritter Avenue
Indianapolis, IN 46219
(317) 355-5069

Kosciusko Community Hospital and Wellness Center
2101 East DuBois Drive
Warsaw, IN 46580
(219) 267-3200

IOWA

Covenant Medical Center
211 East Ridgeway Avenue
Waterloo, IA 50702
(319) 272-2272

Marian Health Center
801 Fifth Street
Sioux City, IA 51102
(712) 279-2579
Offers Phase III at $3.00 per session.

Saint Luke's Health System
2720 Stone Park Boulevard
Sioux City, IA 51104
(712) 279-3808
http://www.siouxlan.com/stlukes

The University of Iowa Hospitals and Clinics
200 Hawkins Drive
Iowa City, IA 52242
(319) 353-8881

KANSAS

Susan B. Allen Memorial Hospital
720 West Central
El Dorado, KS 67042
(316) 322-4517

LOUISIANA

Lake Charles Memorial Hospital
1701 Oak Park Boulevard
Lake Charles, LA 70601
(318) 494-3259

Saint Tammany Parish Hospital
1203 South Tyler Street
Covington, LA 70433
(504) 898-3785

MAINE

Saint Joseph's Healthcare
900 Broadway, Building Three
Bangor, ME 04401
(207) 262-1809

MARYLAND

Dorchester General Hospital
300 Byrn Street
Cambridge, MD 21613
(410) 228-5511

Johns Hopkins Bayview Medical Center
4940 Eastern Avenue
Baltimore, MD 21224
(410) 550-0860

Memorial Hospital
219 South Washington Street
Easton, MD 21601
(410) 822-1000, extension 5208

Peninsula Regional Medical Center
100 East Carroll Street
Salisbury, MD 21801
(410) 543-7026

Saint Agnes HealthCare
900 Canton Avenue
Baltimore, MD 21229
(410) 368-2044

MASSACHUSETTS

Berkshire Medical Center
725 North Street
Pittsfield, MA 01201
(413) 447-3093

Noble Hospital
Cardiopulmonary Rehabilitation
115 West Silver Street
Westfield, MA 01085
(413) 568-2811, extension 5558
Also offers Phase III programs.

MISSOURI

DePaul Health Center
12303 DePaul Drive
Bridgeton, MO 63044
(314) 344-6177

MONTANA

Deaconess Billings Clinic
2800 Tenth Avenue North
Billings, MT 59101
(406) 657-4075

NEBRASKA

Nebraska Health System
982085 Nebraska Medical Center
600 South Forty-second Street
Omaha, NE 68198-2085
(402) 559-9503
http://www.unmc.edu

NEW HAMPSHIRE

Cheshire Medical Center
580 Court Street
Keene, NH 03431
(603) 355-2566

Dartmouth-Hitchcock Medical Center
One Medical Center Drive
Lebanon, NH 03756
(603) 650-5533

NEW MEXICO

Saint Vincent Hospital
Center for Living Well
455 Saint Michael's Drive
Santa Fe, NM 87505
(505) 820-5549

NEW YORK

Beth Israel Medical Center-South
First Avenue at Sixteenth Street
New York, NY 10003
(212) 420-2357

Hudson Valley Hospital Center
1980 Crompond Road
Cortlandt, NY 10567
(914) 734-3810

Jamaica Hospital Medical Center
8900 Van Wyck Expressway
Jamaica, NY 11418
(718) 206-6595

New York Downtown Hospital
New York University Medical Center
170 William Street
New York, NY 10038
(212) 312-5006

Putnam Hospital Center
66 Stoneleigh Avenue
Carmel, NY 10512
(914) 279-5711

NORTH CAROLINA

Duke University Medical Center
Pulmonary Rehabilitation Program
1300 Morrene Road
Durham, NC 27705
(919) 660-6658

North Carolina Baptist Hospital
Medical Center Boulevard
Winston-Salem, NC 27157
(800) 828-2001

University Health Systems
Pitt County Memorial Hospital
2100 Stantonburg Road
Greenville, NC 27835
(252) 816-5736

NORTH DAKOTA

MeritCare Pulmonary Rehabilitation
720 Fourth Street North
Fargo, ND 58122
(701) 234-5659

OHIO

Mount Carmel Health Center
793 West State Street
Columbus, OH 43222
(614) 234-5754

Also has a facility on the east side of the city.

PENNSYLVANIA

Allegheny General Hospital
Cardiac and Pulmonary Rehabilitation Services
320 East North Avenue
Pittsburgh, PA 15212
(412) 359-4662

Sharon Regional Health Systems
"The Lung Center"
740 East State Street
Sharon, PA 16146
(724) 983-3883

University of Pennsylvania
Pulmonary Conditioning
Third Floor, White Building
3400 Spruce Street
Philadelphia, PA 19104
(215) 662-6482

TEXAS

Cardiopulmonary Fitness and Disease Management
338 Lindberg
McAllen, TX 78501
(956) 618-1055

Hillcrest Health System
Getterman Wellness Center
7300 Bosque Boulevard
Waco, TX 76710
(254) 202-3800

Sid Peterson Memorial Hospital
710 Water Street
Kerrville, TX 78028
(830) 896-4200

Warm Springs Rehabilitation System
5101 Medical Drive
San Antonio, TX 78229
(210) 614-9276

UTAH

Cottonwood Hospital
5770 South Third Street East
Murray, UT 84107
(801) 314-2701

VERMONT

Brattleboro Memorial Hospital
17 Belmont Avenue
Brattleboro, VT 05301
(802) 257-8897

VIRGINIA

Lynchburg General Hospital
1901 Tate Springs Road
Lynchburg, VA 24501
(804) 947-4540

Richmond Memorial Hospital
Hanover Medical Park
1300 Westwood Avenue
Richmond, VA 23220
(804) 254-2793

Saint Nicholas Hospital
1601 North Taylor Drive
Sheboygan, WI 53081
(920) 459-4787 or (920) 459-4611

Index

About the Author

MARK JENKINS is the author of several books on health. He co-wrote *The Sports Medicine Bible,* a Book-of-the-Month Club alternate selection. Mark lives year-round on the island of Martha's Vineyard off the coast of Cape Cod, Massachusetts. He travels occasionally to the mainland by ferryboat to fulfill his duties as publishing consultant at the world-renowned Boston Children's Hospital.

Other titles that may interest you . . .

HIGH BLOOD PRESSURE
Practical, Medical, and Spiritual Guidelines for Daily Living with Hypertension

by Mark Jenkins

This book presents basic and essential medical information on the symptoms and causes of high blood pressure, as well as the spiritual aspects of the Twelve Step program that can help those with high blood pressure make positive changes in attitude and behavior to address challenges presented by this disease.

180 pages   Order no. 1368

FINDING THE JOY IN TODAY
Practical Readings for Living with Chronic Illness

by Sefra Kobrin Pizele

These daily meditations address the physical, emotional, and spiritual challenges faced by those who have a chronic illness, helping them regain peace of mind by focusing on the joy to be found in each day.

384 pages   Order no. 5489

CHRONIC ILLNESS AND THE TWELVE STEPS
A Practical Approach to Spiritual Resilience

by Martha Cleveland, Ph.D.

This interpretation of the Twelve Steps integrates beliefs and behaviors that help people cope with chronic illness through a hopeful prophesy and commitment to spiritual wellness.

222 pages   Order no. 1024

THE CHRONIC ILLNESS EXPERIENCE
Embracing the Imperfect Life

by Cheri Register

This book helps those living with an "interminable" illness understand the nonmedical implications (such as the effect the illness has on emotional health, self-image, relationships, work habits, aspirations, and overall outlook on life) and integrate the illness into day-to-day living.

396 pages   Order no. 1023

Hazelden offers titles on a wide range of behavioral and medical chronic illnesses. For price and order information or a free catalog, please call our telephone representatives or visit our Web site at www.hazelden.org

☒ HAZELDEN®

1-800-328-9000   (Toll-Free U.S., Canada, and the Virgin Islands)
1-651-213-4000   (Outside the U.S. and Canada)
1-651-213-4590   (24-Hour Fax)
www.hazelden.org
15251 Pleasant Valley Road • P.O. Box 176
Center City, Minnesota 55012-0176